A VISIT FROM ELIJAH

*An in-depth study and interpretation
of the transition from
Elijah to Elisha
1 Kings Chapters 17-22
2 Kings Chapters 1-2*

Izauh 61®

Copyright 2026 by Harvest of Healing, LLC.

Published 2026.

Printed in the United States of America.

All rights reserved.

No portion of this book may be reproduced, stored in a retrieval system, or transmitted in any form or by any means – electronic, mechanical, photocopy, recording, scanning, or other – except for brief quotations in critical reviews or articles, without the prior written permission of the author.

Softcover ISBN 978-1-965754-14-6
Hardcover ISBN 978-1-965754-15-3
Cover image: Shutterstock

HARVEST OF HEALING, LLC

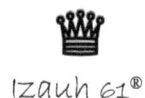

Izauh 61®

Publishing assistance by BookCrafters, Parker, Colorado.
www.bookcrafters.net

INDEX OF CONTENTS

INTRODUCTION 1

OVERVIEW 7

ETYMOLOGY OF KEY WORDS 11

CHAPTER 1
WATER RUNS DRY 17

CHAPTER 2
HELLO GOD, ARE YOU OUT THERE? 28

CHAPTER 3
THE THREAT OF DEATH 45

CHAPTER 4
WHAT'S ALL THE NOISE ABOUT? 51

CHAPTER 5
THE VINEYARD TOO? 58

CHAPTER 6
TAKING POSSESSION OF WHAT IS YOURS 63

CHAPTER 7
IT'S ALL IN YOUR HEAD..73

CHAPTER 8
A WHIRLWIND OF ACTIVITY..78

CHAPTER 9
RAINING MANNA..87

CONCLUSION...95

INTRODUCTION

What if I were to tell you that genetic <u>mutations</u> (I often refer to them as an imprint) are not the root cause of disease? That there is still another layer to the health disruptions that burp out in the form of disease. Would you believe this, or chalk it up as folly?

Mutations are described as the structural faults within the DNA. The spiral staircase called helix becomes damaged in some way, often in many ways, and that damage sends harmful signals to the body that spell out death, decay and disease. Like a piano keyboard with two or three keys that no longer function, or produce a sour tune, so is the damaged DNA signal. The body can only do what it is told and the structure of DNA, the helix, the chromosomes, etcetera make up the broadcasting station the body responds to. Manipulating the body makes little headway when it comes to trying to snuff out the signals that come from damaged DNA. Like a house built on a faulty foundation and building materials that lack quality, eventually things will fall apart.

Genetic imprints, the damages to the DNA strands, were formed by something along the walk of life. They are a result of an action, otherwise they wouldn't exist. Since imprints are not the root issue when it comes to health, what is it that is rocking the boat of good, healthy, complete DNA strands?

Imprints are developed out of recorded information that resides in dirty plasma. Water records vibrations through electrical activity and everything that exists is a result of a vibration, singular or multiple in nature. Building cells on the records held by the water (plasma), where every infection, sound, action, smell, color, and so forth that was encountered is held, it is no surprise DNA strands are damaged by this point in time. Polluted plasma equals structurally weak or damaged DNA. The library of prerecorded information the plasma is encoded with becomes the structural foundation for DNA strands. When plasma carries contamination, the entirety of the DNA structure including chromosomes will be polluted and damaged. So how is this polluted water cleaned?

To erase the genetic imprints, plasma must go through a cleansing process. This cleansing process could be compared to the cycles of a washing machine. Water fills the tub, agitates the clothing back and forth or around and around, drains the water out through a spin cycle and then follows all of this with a rinse cycle. Any cells that contain damaged DNA strands will die off (or at least be cleansed) during a proper cleansing process, and new cells will be made with healthy DNA strands once the plasma is clean. While the process is a slow one, taking up to 7 years to complete, it holds a promise of few or no encounters with disease or crippling decay for the remaining years. Follow the guidelines written many years ago for health and a healthy life is what you will produce.

What I share is not only what I have experienced but what I discovered in chapters and verses held in the Holy Bible near the end of my personal "visit from Elijah," Elijah being the process the body orchestrates to clean the plasma and eliminate the curses cast down upon us from our ancestors which are the collection of contamination that produces damaged DNA. First, be aware that Elijah comes unannounced and unexpected, in part because people have no concept of how to identify Elijah. There are no premade arrangements by human effort or the mind for this visitation. A bigger issue is the ability to identify the fact that Elijah was lost through time. Now is the time for Elijah's identity to be resurrected!

This publication will unfold what I call the Elijah Healing. The Elijah Healing must be applied if a person desires to accomplish "salvation." Yes, I said salvation. What is salvation exactly? Salvation means rescue. Rescue from what? The disruptions in your health that trouble you. Those genetic imprints left behind by ancestors that reside in the blood, often called a curse in biblical stories. There are numerous health disturbances a person could be rescued from, but Elijah's visitation is focused on the foundations of good health and removing the embedded recordings that repeatedly play in the body and build damaged DNA strands, damaged chromosomes, and eventually unfold as disease.

To interrupt the Elijah Healing with various forms of common physical treatment or therapy, described in the stories as consulting Baal, will only delay the process of eliminating what the body identifies as harmful. The body can eliminate a measure of chemical pollution at any given time, but it is the continual intake of harmful substances, legal or illegal, that interfere with the elimination of the imprints left by ancestors that result in disease. Like adding water and fuel to the same fire, you make little headway. Like all cellular constructed beings, the physical body will attempt to eliminate, through its own means, the disruptions that hinder its cycle of life. The body is far more complex than what science has discovered to date or is willing to talk about. Without the Elijah Healing, the human body experiences decay and death, sometimes in a manner that is not at all pleasant.

When I began the journey through the jungle of deadly health issues, I did not realize there would be one specific layout of a story within the Holy Bible that described exactly what I was (and had been) experiencing. During an ordinary chapter and verse review, I came to 1 Kings and the story of Elijah. As I read the story that I had read many times before, the full interpretation unfolded before my eyes. I was in awe of how I had been led through a jungle of deadly health concerns and yet pop out at the opposite side of the journey in better physical health than what I was born with. All a response to unknowingly following the steps laid out within the story of Elijah. The medical industry receives no credit for the successful recovery I have experienced. Now I have tangible, hopefully believable evidence that what I experienced was real, had a divine purpose, and can be experienced by others. I remain amazed. I shared the details of my journey through the jungle of troubling and sometimes deadly health encounters in my book *Home-Made Answers for Cancer and Life Altering Disease*, published in 2024.

Is this process and recovery for every person on earth? Possibly, yet not likely. I believe there are details yet to be discovered that pertain to the intricate structural process of DNA, and male and female structural DNA differences held within the chromosomes. There is a component that is built into the blood that uniquely sets a group of people apart. This specific group may make it through their individual jungle of health concerns with the application of the Elijah Healing wherein someone without this unique DNA quality may not. Any resulting change in the DNA and manifestation of health is dependent upon the level of contamination in the plasma and the level of discipline the individual applies through the process. Please do not misunderstand, this plasma cleansing process is not easy and requires 24/7, 365 disciplines for at least seven years. Given that, I am hopeful that a shift in the chemical elements that reside in the cosmos will become a more prevalent helpmate to those who take on the Elijah Healing assignment. (See previous publications: <u>Living by the Light of the Moon</u>, published in 2024, and <u>Healing the Heart</u>, published in 2025)

A WORD OF CAUTION: Anyone who is on a life-dependent medication will be challenged beyond measure with the Elijah Healing process. While medical intervention may be necessary at times and to various degrees, to use such intervention during the Elijah Healing, a "less is more" approach would be best. Each case is certainly different, and good judgment is always a must. The Elijah Healing process takes up to seven years when a person is not on any form of chemical assistance, replacement or therapy. For example, if a person is on thyroid replacement medication in response to having the thyroid surgically removed, extreme caution should be administered during all phases of the Elijah Healing. All chemicals ingested, applied to the body, inhaled, etc., should be removed under the direction of a professional, when necessary, during the initial phase of the Elijah Healing process. Otherwise, there is a great risk in becoming very ill and simply spinning your wheels, not gaining any ground in recovery. The goal is to cleanse the toxic plasma out of the body and any dose of toxic substance added to the body during the process can simply delay the desired outcome. Personally, I take no prescription drugs, use natural household cleansers, sleep and dress in natural fabrics, and it has taken me nearly seven years to get through my journey. Even with all that in place, parts of the journey seemed at times unbearable. If someone feels they should or could go through the Elijah Healing process, it would be advised to have a mentor.

OVERVIEW

The first 16 chapters of 1 Kings reports the death of David and that Solomon takes the position of king where he begins construction of the temple. Solomon enters into a business agreement with Egypt through his marriage to Pharoah's daughter. Pharoah's daughter lives with Solomon <u>until</u> (Chapter 3, verse 1) he finished building the temple. Interesting fact. It appears Pharoah's daughter was an avenue for a business connection for Solomon and once the assigned business project was complete, Pharoah's daughter was released from her assignment. The biblical story not only references the use of the world's systems (Egypt) for an assigned time, but also marriage relationships. A clear picture of marriage being an access for business transactions is woven into the story. These details put an interesting twist on our current day view of what a marriage is.

Solomon gains favor with God and receives wisdom in response to that favor. How does Solomon gain this favor? He must be doing something specific to receive this favor. Taking into consideration that the temple is technically our physical body, Solomon must be doing something to care for his body that was not necessarily common or popular in the day. He had something or did something that others did not. Was the Elijah Healing a part of Solomon's lifestyle?

The parable in Chapter 3 of the two prostitutes with newborns describes situations where two similar "acts of service" (where *something is being sold to you that satisfies the flesh) produce a response in the flesh (baby boy). One flesh response (baby boy) causes the death of the sonship status (one baby dies), yet that particular "act of service" steals the components (baby) that continues to have life within it. In biblical stories women often represent spirit activity, meaning things that are unseen yet have a measure of influence. This story warns of a form of physically stimulating, or pleasurable situations which will result in the position of being a "son" to die off. Gaining the title of Son must be more challenging than we've been led to believe. This story is not about intimate relations but about soothing the body through a means that eliminates pain or sickness, something that brings relief like an aspirin or Rx would. There is a simple explanation to this stimulation or pleasuring of the flesh found in some, not all, medical treatments or therapies. Medical treatments are specifically directed at relieving discomforts of the flesh.*

Continuing the move through the chapters of 1 Kings, we observe Solomon's power to establish the lost temple, with the temple being a reference point for a healthy physical body. I doubt anyone would argue with the fact that today some measure of health within our physical bodies has been lost. My body is the temple.... Different things contribute to the construction, which tells us there is not one pill, or exercise, or diet that brings the physical body back into its proper function. Multiple building materials are required.

Fast forward through a few chapters where we begin to see various forces come in and out of the picture. Forces are labeled as Kings or Queens, powerful rulers that are over the people. Chapter 10 introduces the Queen of Sheba. In this chapter we learn that 1) spices; 2) precious stones; 3) food; and 4) attire, all contribute to Solomon's assignment (the ability to construct your temple with the use of wisdom) and that these items and acts described will influence the appearance of the physical body (verses 6-7).

In Chapter 11 the story unfolds with the unfaithful acts of Solomon. Foreign women (meaning those who live a different lifestyle or have a different belief system) seem to be an attraction for Solomon. A preference that his father, King David, had. God strictly instructs Solomon in verse 2 to not join in business relationships ("Marriage") with foreign women because of the powerful influence their lifestyle and beliefs would have on him. This part of the Solomon story is not a reference for casting judgment upon joining with someone who has a different skin color but a warning to not join with those who live life outside of the Commands God has given when you are an "Israelite." Such unequal unions become burdensome and can produce offspring with genes that war against each other.

The Israelites begin to grumble and complain about the long list of "do this" and "don't do that" that comes with maintaining the bodily temple (Chapter 12). The Israelites begin acting like rebellious teenagers and trouble in the form of judgments, meaning consequences for your actions, begins to sprout up (Chapter 13, verses 11-34).

Various kings (ruling forces) come and go, and Judah finds itself in some troublesome situations. Judah is known for having strayed from the origins of Israelite blood and this rebellion of sorts causes generation after generation to decline in health. One important thing the bloodline of Judah is known for are our internal cleansing components when the Commands (rules) are properly followed, as seen throughout the story of Jesus, who has "cleansing blood." The details of this unique quality in Judah blood are described in detail throughout the chapters and verses in this publication. Some of the interpretations are challenging to follow and can be quite lengthy in the development of the picture the Scriptures attempt to present. Many biblical stories sprinkle nuggets of information through many books, chapters and verses making it time consuming and challenging to connect all the dots. Some interpretations are easy to spell out. It is the explanation of how I arrived at the interpretation that becomes tricky. My advice is, when something seems vague, stop and ask for assistance from your assigned source of higher power.

Select your favorite translation of the Holy Bible and turn to 1 Kings, Chapter 17. As you read the Chapters within this publication, follow along with each chapter and verse in the bible. Without the accompaniment of the bible, you will likely become lost in what I attempt to describe. With these few details outlined, we can now proceed to the steps required for an Elijah Healing journey that leads to a transformation into Elisha. Let's begin.

ETYMOLOGY OF KEY WORDS

First and foremost is the value of understanding the origins of names. An easy Google search for "etymology of (name)" will give you a brief history of where and how a particular name originated. Any teaching without the exposure of the true meaning and foundations of a name or title is comparable to babbling.

For example, mountain, valley, stream and spring represent specific bladder, gallbladder, spleen and kidney meridians (the electrical highways and chakra points discussed in From Antichrist to I AM, published in 2022). Streams and rivers can also represent the blood vessels and veins that carry blood and plasma through our body.

<u>Abel-Meholah</u>: Stream or brook + dancing; (meridians – where the energy flows. Specific rhythmic movement)

<u>Ahab</u>: Brother; father (ancestors; genetic bloodline)

<u>Ahaziah</u>: Seize, grasp, possession (those who God has possession of – specific DNA structure)

<u>Aphek</u>: Channel, pipe or tube; confinement of the streaming of liquid

<u>Aram</u>: High region; to be high

Asa: To suffer harm or mischief; healer or physician

Asherah: She (spirit/energy) who treads the sea (sea is a meridian. Example: Conception Vessel (CV) 6 is called the Sea of Energy located in the region of the naval.)

Azubah: To leave or forsake; desolation

Baal: Owner or lord (what lords over you; what rules your decisions or actions)

Baal-zebub: Lord of the flies (flies attract to a decaying carcass and/or dung)

Ben-Hadad: Son of a particular house + noise, to cause a commotion

Benjamin: Son of my right hand

Beer-Sheba: Well of the oath or well of seven

Beit-El: House of God

Chariot: Cart; wheeled vehicle (wheels are the chakras as described by Ezekiel). A jaw is compared to a chariot in traditional Chinese medicine acupuncture.

Chenaanah: Synchronize or give up individual leanings to unite as a group; humbled; to bend the knee. Submit

Cherith (Brook or Wadi): Community of misfits; off the main stream; repeated circular motion, designated region; instrument of war; shared cultural identity (misfits would indicate a disruption in proper meridian activity.)

<u>Damascus</u>: Well-watered place/land

<u>Dogs</u>: Those who are a part of the (God's) family but do not adhere to the laws, instead they follow the commands of man – the world. Many dogs are also known to eat anything, and sometimes a lot of whatever is in front of them.

<u>Ekron</u>: Barren or barrenness; pluck or uprooting; extermination

<u>Elijah (expanded)</u>: The most common definitions are Strength of Yah; to be strong; my God is the supreme God. Going a little deeper I found that Eli means "to go up," my God. There are also several descriptions that relate to a yoke of childish behavior, spoiled. This description connects to emotional behavior. A tree's leafage is another description. This can represent the family tree, leafage being ancestors spread out over time. Leafage on trees appears during a specific time of year and then later in the year those leaves can fall off, representing the cyclical activity of cell die-off and duplication. The genetic imprints will become active for a cycle and then they quiet themselves for a cycle – round and round they go. But the most interesting description is "water-course + healing." With this, the role of Elijah is carved out through the water/plasma status so that when clean, brings a healing, not only of genetic imprints but also of emotional disruptions, and proper function of the meridian highways. Elijah is the only character in the Holy Bible that is identified as a Tishbite. Tishbite means one who is self-sufficient, frugal in his ways. Self-sufficient reflects how the body can and will heal itself.

<u>Elisha</u>: Salvation through/by God

<u>Ezion Geber</u>: Skeletal structure; strength; backbone of a man

<u>Gilead</u>: Perpetual fountain; heap of testimony; to roll

Gilgal: Heaping, whirling, rolling, bowl or basin, circle or time, age

Hazael: He who sees God; God has seen. Approach or negation; window to see or experience

Imla: Cycle of harvest, storage and redistribution; wither or weaken; filling of gold with jewels; fullness

Israel: One who wrestles with God; struggles

Jehoram: Jehovah is exalted (high)

Jehoshaphat: God has judged - decided

Jehu: Jehovah is He. Wailing, muffled groaning, labored utterance

Jericho: Respite, relief + fragrance; city of the Moon

Jezebel: Without honor; no "husband" (lack of connection/union with cosmic activity; a lack of Holy Spirit guidance; to act and make decisions solely on circumstances.)

Jezreel: Seed, offspring, sowing, seat of strength, scatter; he will be sown of God

Jordan: Descend; to flow down; down under

Judah: Worthy of praise; splendor; glory

Kir-hareseth: Wall; fortress; stronghold

Kishon: Lay bait, line, snare, place of ensnarement

Living Water: Internal hydration produced by the body by the means of Heavenly Gases (oxygen) and hydrogen from fresh bread. The movement of clean plasma that brings the cleansing resulting in healing/health.

<u>Manna</u>: Connects to the chemical elements from heaven and the mouth. Coriander seed is mentioned which has a fragrance (fresh breath) and is described as being white (a whitening agent for the teeth). It is not necessary to eat or use coriander seed, it is simply a reference to the protection given to the mouth, teeth and gums. The mouth an entry point for chemical elements that descend from the heavens during nighttime hours. Manna is the term used to reference that the tissues, gums and teeth will be used during the Elijah Healing process by providing the necessary nutrition and sustenance through chemical elements and electrical activity housed in the teeth.

<u>Micaiah</u>: Who is like God. (son of Imlah)

<u>Moab</u>: Mental footing; father; to decide; water of the father

<u>Mount Carmel</u>: Plantation, garden, vineyard, orchard, fruitful field; what comes through the "seed." (Must eat an abundance of fresh fruit through the Elijah Healing.)

<u>Naboth</u>: Fruit; sprout; fertility

<u>Nebat</u>: To look to, regard or consider; expectation

<u>Nimshi</u>: Rescued from danger

<u>Obadiah</u>: To serve the Lord – servant of the Lord; to work as a slave or hired expert

<u>Ophir</u>: Riches, gathering mark for wealth; inner wealth or wisdom

<u>Prophet</u>: A prophet represents the response the meridians take as they are directed by the Heavenly Gases within the body. A messaging system that is directed by "God" and runs the systems of the body, similar in likeness to the intricate messaging system of chromosomes. This messaging system can also produce insight,

revelation and/or predictions that are present within. The cosmic atmosphere holds records of past events and those records can be read by one who is called a prophet. What has been is what shall be. Life is cyclical in nature. At times, prophet is a reference to the genes held within the blood that reach back to ancestors that followed the Commands (Laws of the Universe) for good health. Those prophets, sound bites from ancestor cells that are healthy, will resurrect from their quiet or dead state once the more recent, contaminated cells are removed or shut off. A sort of clearing the dance floor and they will come alive concept.

Ramot: Height; elevations

Samaria: To keep or guard, watching

Shafat: To judge, governor; a ruling in a penal sense; ordinance, custom or manner

Shilhi: To send or let go like in the firing of an arrow or missile; outstretching; discharge from service

Sideon: Hunter, fish or game, net, stronghold; provisions, food

Sodom: Deal violently with; destroy + field

Syria: Straight or upright; decisive progression, to make things right; a walk or a going; happiness; tree (family tree)

Tarshish: White dove or Holy Spirit

Tishbite: Homesteader, frugal or self-sufficient; returnee

Widow: to separate; to be empty

Zarephath: Smelt, refine, test

Zedekiah: Just; righteous

CHAPTER I
1 KINGS, CHAPTER 17

WATER RUNS DRY

1 Kings beginning with Chapter 17:

<u>Verses 1-7</u>: The scene takes place in Gilead (a continuously flowing fountain), where Elijah speaks to Ahab regarding the removal of dew and rain for a specified increment of time. A wadi is a dry riverbed that flows with water only during or after heavy rain and is usually dry most of the year. The human body, with respect to the plasma, should have this same periodic flowing that is "dry most of the year" concept and water being in abundance at specified increments of time. Considering normal seasonal components, summer heat is the time of year when rivers dry up or water levels decline, and water evaporates easily. During the hot, dry summer months many creeks and streams become dry, allowing fungi or bacteria to die-off. This natural occurring process is a comparison to the water within the body, the plasma. The existing plasma must decrease or be removed from the body so fresh, clean water can take its place. The vibrations of viruses, bacteria and other microorganisms will attach to the plasma and be removed from the body when the Elijah Healing process is followed.

Elijah receives instruction from the Lord to leave his location and move eastward to a place where he can be in <u>isolation, or secluded</u>, described as hide/hiding. This area of seclusion is to be near the wadi

Cherith. A descriptive word for Cherith is misfit. It appears the pathways for plasma transportation by means of veins or blood vessels are experiencing distress. These distressed vein and blood vessel pathways connect to the Jordan. Jordan has a meaning of going down, descend. There are a couple of ways to view the name Jordan. Jordan can reference the location within the body, interior, down under the surface. Jordan can also represent a situation where one would lose their status or footing, instability or loss of credibility.

Instruction continues to be given to Elijah. Elijah is told that he will "drink from the wadi." Think about this for a moment. If Cherith has a meaning that consists of something being out of sorts, then being instructed to drink from that wadi gives a notion that the hydration the body is receiving from the plasma has an element that creates a disruption in the form of what is described as a misfit. Could this misfit be the genetic imprints? To drink is a reference to an assigned, current situation. This is seen in Jesus requesting that "this cup" (His assignment to be tortured and hung on a cross) be taken from Him.

Elijah is told that his body will receive its hydration from the wadi and that his food would be sourced by the ravens. What meaning do the ravens have? Birds are viewed as things that move through the air, those things that are felt yet not always seen. The wind is a good example of this. You can see the result of wind, but you do not see the wind itself. The symbolism of a raven stretches back over time and cultures. Descriptions for a raven would include: transformation, a bridge between the physical and spiritual. In Norse mythology the raven is seen as one's thoughts or memory activity. Celtic lore labels the raven as a symbol of fate, prophesy and the mysteries of life and death. Multiple descriptions exist and most descriptions depend *upon the theme of the story at hand. In this story, the ravens are the memory activity held in the cells. If the plasma contamination is not addressed, it will result in death in some form or another.*

Elijah follows the instructions given him and sets up his tent by the wadi Cherith. Appears Elijah has found his new living space and is prepared for the water within the body to begin its work. Let's put a little different spin on what "to live by" could really being saying. What if Elijah wasn't really living "next to" the wadi but adjusted his life to live "according to" the ways of the wadi? Something to consider.

Notice Elijah ate bread and meat in the morning and in the evening (1 Kings 17:6). There is no indication of a meal at mid-day, or noon. I will emphasize here that meat is often a reference to nourishment, not animal flesh. During the Elijah Healing process there should be no consumption of animal flesh for at least the first several months. Considering the chemical reaction the Elijah Healing is to achieve, I cannot advise eating meat, animal flesh, in the morning. Sorry, no bacon or breakfast sausage! Animal flesh is only permitted on specific days in alignment with the moon cycle and is to be avoided, along with all animal products, on Sabbath days. Eating meat outside of the specified times can result in damage to the internal mechanisms of the physical body over time and is a disruption to the production of gases that initiate cleansing inside the body. It is the best advice to remove all animal products and flesh until all genetic imprints are removed.

The reference to bread is two-fold. FRESHLY-made bread provides hydrogen and gluten. Any bread held over to the next day without freezing loses a measure of the hydrogen and gluten influence. Hydrogen plus oxygen produces water, even inside the body. There should be very little or better yet, no water consumption during the Elijah Healing. Reducing water intake may need to be a gradual process for some but the goal is to eliminate drinking water as a source of hydration. No, you will not dehydrate. Hydration will come from consuming fresh fruits and from the hydrogen-oxygen combination provided when eating fresh bread.

In the story of King David and the death of his infant son born to him by Bathsheba, King David was offered bread during his time of grieving over his son. King David refuses the bread stating a curse would be upon him if he ate bread prior to sunset. Eating bread during the hours between sunrise and sunset (some translations say dawn and dusk) could awaken the curse (genetic imprint) cast upon (inherited) you by your ancestors. It is possible that eating bread outside of the guidelines given could create other health issues. When I stopped eating bread and pasta during sunlit hours, my energy level increased and the necessity to take a nap in the afternoon ceased. In biblical stories the word 'curse' is used to describe the contaminated genetic soup received by an individual at conception. Once the contaminated genetic recordings are activated, your life will display a "curse" or record of the ancestor's sin. Bread is to be eaten at dawn and dusk. Continue reading.

Given time, waterways will dry up in summer heat as a result of evaporation and the lack of rain. (More on rain in Chapter 9, Raining Manna). This illustration also unfolds within the body. Reduce the water intake, allow the water/plasma to be reduced and contamination to be removed making room for clean, fresh water/plasma.

Verses 8-11: Now Elijah experiences various levels of testing through the need to restrict or eliminate foods. Today, the list of food that is to be avoided is quite lengthy. This is not a one week or one month situation. This is a required act of restraint that lasts for at least four to five years of this seven-year journey. As time progresses during this food restriction phase, many foods once thought to be a "must have" are no longer appealing. The internal body can be very slow at accomplishing the entirety of elimination of curses (contaminated genetic imprints) and rebuilding the body with new, healthy cells. Your appetite will be tested and will eventually adjust. Food restrictions are put into place not only as a test of how well a person can refrain from physical desires but also to allow the chemicals that govern the function of the body to be adjusted. More detail is given on the diet restrictions required in <u>Home-Made Answers for Cancer and Life Altering Disease</u>, published in 2024.

Elijah receives word that a widow (to separate or be empty) woman will be his means of support through this part of the journey. Why a widow woman? One meaning for widow is to separate. Acts of isolation are valuable during the Elijah Healing process. In the current days and times people are very active and over-exposed to various situations, people, environments, and so on that influence the process the cells are attempting to go through. Remember the test days when you were in school? How the room that accommodated those taking a test needed to be quiet and with no interruptions? This same quiet, no interruptions, is what the body requires to properly process and/or eliminate the contamination and misinformation it has received over the years.

Elijah arrives at his destination (Zarephath) of isolation and testing in connection with food (Sideon) and encounters a gate. A gate is a reference to an access point. Gates are also specific meridian points in the body. For example: the Spirit Gate that feeds the heart (H7). A city represents a place overseen by a governing power that people reside within. Behold, a widow woman was there gathering sticks (branches from the family tree). Elijah gets the widow woman's attention and says: "Bring me, I pray you, a little water in a vessel, so I can drink." (<u>Midline Meridians are called Conception Vessel and Governing Vessel.</u>) The widow woman follows Elijah's request and as she goes to get the water Elijah inserts a second request for a piece of bread "in your hand." Two things are at play in this scene. Water, which would be fresh, or contamination-free plasma through the means of isolation and diet restrictions, and bread that is made by hand. No bread machines! There is an energetic electrical component that is interwoven into bread dough when it is kneaded by hand. Knowing how many other things work, it seems the distribution of this hands-on component activates some chemical, nutrient or gas related element in the bread.

<u>Verses 12-16</u>: Some peculiar details are held in these verses. Ground grain (wheat) combined with a little olive oil will initiate a process for the ancestral contamination (genetic imprints) to die off. Interesting. It sure beats many of the medical science approaches of today. Wait, do they even have an answer for eliminating genetic imprints? As of the writing of this book, no they do not, as far as those that are disclosed, anyway.

Moving on through these verses, Elijah tells the widow woman that the bread and oil will need to be consumed until "the day the Lord sends <u>rain</u> upon the earth." Does this statement mean literal rain? Doubtful, since the earth receives occasional rain to this day. There is a hint that chemical elements are involved. What is present in the clouds will descend to the earth. Rain is a reference to the transfer of chemical elements from the Heavens (clouds) down to earth. The day and time we currently live in is the beginning of "the day of the Lord." (2 Peter 3:8)

Will there be a shift that brings a new combination of chemical elements (identified as rain in the story) to the earth that will assist the body in elimination of the contamination we see today as genetic imprints or even DNA and chromosome defects? What a glorious day that would be!

The bread is unleavened bread made by hand, often these days called a tortilla. The first serving of bread will feed the Elijah Healing process, and after that the physical body is fed. Basically, when you eat the tortilla(s), the first tortilla eaten will provide the required chemical combination for the body to rid itself of genetic imprints. If you so choose, a second tortilla can be eaten, but it only serves as a satisfaction for the appetite, not contributing to the healing process. The bread is to be eaten with a small amount of olive oil. The first nine months of the Elijah Healing experience I did not eat salt, condiments or leavening agents. I ate my hand made bread with olive oil. After nine months I added salt to my olive oil. Once the plasma is clean, salt aids in keeping the plasma clean of unwanted debris. Salt is also important for the electrical activity that is to be present in the chromosomes. More information on salt is found in Chapter 8.

According to Exodus 27:20, the bread is to be eaten with olive oil, so the light (I call this light Star Dust), will always be present. The verse states, in part: ...command the children of Israel to bring you pure olive oil, beaten (crushed) <u>for the light</u>, to cause the lamp to burn always.

For human life to remain on the earth, the cosmic activity will provide a measure of electromagnetics and chemical elements. Otherwise, human life would become non-existent moving at the current rates we are witnessing in disease and death. Once the cosmic activity completes the shift that it is currently orchestrating, it will become necessary for humans to position themselves through consumption of fresh bread, wearing natural fabrics, avoiding chemicals, limiting stressful activity, etc. to have the proper measure of Heavenly Gases that keep the body in a healthy state of existence.

If you witnessed the majestic sunrise of December 9th that was displayed over the Colorado sky, you saw the predicted change that was presented in living color across the heavens. It was truly one of the most beautiful displays of color I have ever seen, and I only saw a photo of it. Color is a result of what? Vibration! The "New Heavens" are taking shape and that change will make its way to the earth. <u>Isaiah 65:17</u>: "For I will create a new heaven and a new earth; the past events will not be remembered or come to mind." (HCS)

The widow woman did according to Elijah's request, and she and her house ate for <u>many days</u>. The instruction here is to eat in your own home. Eating food prepared by restaurants will cause interruptions in the Elijah Healing process and you could end up in a worse health position than what you started with. "Many days" means eating the bread will need to take place over an extended period. I am currently in year 7 of my Elijah Healing process and I still eat fresh bread and drink grape juice each evening at or shortly after dusk.

Continue to eat fresh bread with olive oil and sea salt even after the designated years for cleaning the damaged DNA strands is complete. "According to the word of the Lord" means this activity (eating fresh bread and drinking grape juice) is a Universal Law.

<u>Verses 17-18</u>: There will be periods of time when your physical body is knocking on death's door. You feel it, you look it, you sense it. In my personal experience, my lungs were influenced, producing a cough

and yellow-green phlegm. My lungs were purging contaminated fluid that had backed up into my chest cavity. It was ugly, it was unsettling, and with a double genetic imprint for lung cancer I cannot help but think the lung contamination would have overtaken me had I discontinued the restrictions of the Elijah Healing. The best advice is to stay focused and do not wander from the dietary restrictions. The intake of fresh bread with olive oil is a must. Concord grape juice provides necessary chromium and 2-4 ounces, maximum, is what should be consumed with the bread. Too much fluid in the body diminishes the ability of the gases to do their work. Breath represents the necessary chemical elements (Heavenly Gases), not just oxygen, to sustain life.

For the genetic imprints to be removed, the body brings them to the surface, and they present a symptom. I went through several and various symptomatic experiences. The key to success, is to not waiver in the application of the Elijah Healing. Stick with it!

Now the widow woman questions her connection to Elijah. Then she closes her question with "you man of God." Man is reference to the physical body, flesh. The reference to God is indicative of the combination of chemical elements, electricity, cosmic activity and all the other wonders that are present in or around the body. Elijah must have had a noticeable essence about him. Considering the word widow means to separate, it can be safely assumed that this verse is telling us that when a person separates themselves (from being amongst the crowd or taking part in worldly events), the continual presence of God (ability to maintain a measure of the chemical elements in and around the physical body; successful upkeep of the aura around you) is what makes them different from others. The presence (of God) evaporates or dissipates in crowds and noise.

Again, the widow woman asks a question in an accusatory manner. She wants to know if Elijah came to her to cause her body to remember, or bring to the surface, the iniquities that her body carries. The iniquities would create a situation where the position of "sonship" is removed. In other words, this woman cannot figure out why this Elijah Healing is causing her such great misery in her health. She knows that this level of misery can cause any measure of Star Dust to escape and the position of "son" to be removed. She's probably thinking things are moving in the wrong direction! Iniquity is a classification of sin (an immoral act or deviation from righteousness) and that sin is being brought to the surface by being made evident through symptoms.

<u>Verses 19-24</u>. Elijah takes the son and carries him to his bed where Elijah stretches himself upon (or over) the child three times while praying for the life of the son to be restored.

The Elijah Healing brings the Heavenly Gases (breath) that restore the status of sonship. Your bed will become a safe space, and a bed should support one person, not two or more. Naps and ample rest are required for the activity taking place with respect to the cells. The reference to three times 1) a limit is set; 2) reaching to three generations; or 3) the duration of the first three years of the Elijah Healing is taking care of restoring a sonship status and assisting your offspring in the process. To 'stretch' references an act of reaching beyond; reaching beyond the widow woman and touching even the child (descendants) of the woman. A woman has the power to assist in healing damaged DNA for her offspring when it comes to any inherited DNA the child receives. A child must tend to their own Elijah Healing to correct DNA damage that is self-inflicted or left unaddressed by ancestors. Note that Elijah asked for the child's "life" to come into him "again." The life (soul) is removed when the plasma *becomes overly contaminated and full of toxic debris and in turn depletes the Heavenly Gases required for life. The Elijah Healing is the only thing that will resurrect the life/soul by removal of the inherited contamination (sin).*

Elijah's request for the life to be restored to the son is heard and answered. The son being brought out of the 'chamber' is equivalent to there being no more sickbeds. The widow woman is astounded. Now she is convinced that the Elijah Healing comes from God.

CHAPTER 2
1 KINGS, CHAPTER 18

HELLO GOD, ARE YOU OUT THERE?

Verses 1-2: These verses mention that Elijah had been through a period where God's voice had become silent. Elijah is not hearing anything until the third year. The third year of what? The third year of the restrictions in place with respect to bread, water and not hanging out with the crowd of friends he has. It is clear that the process for a complete transformation in health through the Elijah Healing is a slow one.

Now Elijah is given the command to appear before Ahab. Ahab means brother or father which equates to ancestors. It appears this Elijah Healing is going to confront the genetic corruption left behind by ancestors. The famine in Samaria indicates the lack of an act that would protect the body through removal of harmful habits. Samaria means to guard or keep. Humans have failed to guard the health of their body through restricting food intake, particularly on specific days of the moon's cycle. Improper food intake is the #1 harmful habit. Cells begin to die off when there is proper limited caloric intake. I do not suggest or support removing all food and/or drink for extended periods of time. Extended fasting can do more harm than good. The body must have a way to produce the necessary gases for the Elijah Healing process to continue.

Bread was the staple food and when fresh bread is missing from the diet, the cells can become polluted by the debris encountered during any typical day. Those unattended debris cause damage to the DNA, cells, chromosomes and pass through the bloodline. The bread must be eaten daily to assist in cleansing the debris out of the blood and protecting the plasma from harmful influences. In my experience, as best as I could follow the events, the first three years the Elijah Healing took care of the oldest inherited cellular debris and imprints. From the third year until the fifth or sixth year, the Elijah Healing begins to move through the inherited imprints that are from your parents and grandparents, the more recent imprints, those that are from three to four generations back.

<u>Deuteronomy 5:9 (HCS)</u>: You must not bow down to them or worship them, because I, the Lord your God, am a jealous God, punishing the children for the fathers' sin to the third and fourth generations of those who hate Me, but showing faithful love to a thousand generations to those who love Me and keep My commands.

Three and four generations can bring with it a lot of toxic debris to unload and again, it can present numerous symptoms, all dependent upon what the actions, words and lifestyle of the ancestors were. There are no secrets when God is involved in cleaning house! What grandma or grandpa did, whether it was smoking, drinking alcoholic beverages, eating poorly, or numerous other things, will come out through you in the form of a troubling symptom!

<u>Verses 3-6</u>: Ahab sends a text message to Obadiah (that which serves the Lord; servant). Obadiah respected the Commands for living (Laws of the Universe) and protected 100 prophets while Jezebel was on a rampage. What are prophets? Messages delivered that come directly from God. Going out on a limb here, I suggest that 100

prophets are symbolic of healthy cellular recordings from ancestors of 10 or more generations back (1,000 generations as referenced in the Deuteronomy verse) that lived by the Commands. How did Obadiah protect the prophets? With bread, respecting seasonal cycles, following food restrictions, and I say the reference to water is speaking of the plasma. When there is too much water in the body the electrical activity is hindered, and the excess fluid moves to and parks in various parts of the body. When water collects in the region of the chest, the lungs become influenced. It is doubtful people of the days and times referenced in the Holy Bible drank water for the reason described above and, there were limited freshwater wells available. Grape juice or other fruit juices would have been the drink of choice.

I need to bring attention to Numbers 6:3. This verse describes the law for a Nazarite (to separate oneself or consecrate). The HCS version of the verse states: … he is to abstain from wine and beer. He must not drink vinegar made from wine or from beer. He must not drink any <u>grape juice</u> or eat fresh grapes or raisins. The NKJ version of the verse states: He shall separate himself from wine and strong drink and shall drink no vinegar of wine, or vinegar of strong drink, neither shall he drink any <u>liquor of grapes</u>, nor eat moist grapes, or dried. Emphasis is added to the references of grape juice and liquor of grapes. This verse is a good example of how translation from one language to another can throw a kink in the true meaning. With respect to the Elijah Healing process, I began drinking organic Concord Grape Juice at the beginning of my Elijah Healing and still drink it to this day with my fresh bread. I have consumed more grape juice in the past 7 years than I had in the total years I have had my feet on soil. I gradually eliminated drinking of water in about the third or fourth year. Grape juice was my drink of choice. However, I did not eat whole grapes or raisins. I suggest the translation should read the <u>pulp</u> (skins and seeds as well) from grapes should be avoided. Grape juice has been a lifeline for me and at times I felt I couldn't drink enough of it. Grape juice is what accompanies the fresh bread.

Let's zero in on Jezebel. Jezebel means there is no husband, and no husband equates to no encounters with the cosmic activity. Proper cosmic connection can activate the prerecorded cellular messages from ancestors called "prophet." This prophetic download is a result of a connection to the soundwaves in the atmosphere that trigger the cell to play its message. Messages can play out in dreams or real-life encounters that hold an interpretation of a deeper meaning and purpose. Without the electrical cosmic connection called husband, there are no true prophets. What has been spilled out through "prophetic words" (often within a religious congregation) is often missing vital information and distributes mere bits and pieces of a much larger picture, if it contains any truth at all. This is the difference between false prophets and true prophets as described in Ezekiel 13:4 and Lamentations 2:14. The lack of contact with the cosmic activity the bible calls husband, interferes with one's ability to hear directly from God. The removal of the husband connection is called Jezebel.

Obadiah is sent on a mission involving the wadi and fountains of water. There are several meridian points in the body identified with various names for water. Stream, brook, rushing, spring, and sea all reference meridian points. These meridians play a role in the production and movement of electricity in the body, and ultimately the pump that keeps the water moving

Grass is a reference to the flesh. <u>Psalm 37:2 (HCS)</u>: For they wither quickly like grass and wilt like tender green plants. There is an act to save the power within the flesh. The verses reference horses and mules. Horses are a symbol of power, and a mule is known to "carry the load," a burden. Some form of burden that is afflicting the flesh appears to need attention.

Ahab and Obadiah split up and move in different directions.

<u>Verses 7-14</u>: Obadiah is moving along on his journey, and he meets a man he thought to be Elijah. Obadiah inquires if the person he was seeing was really Elijah. Elijah responds, it is I and then instructs Obadiah to go and get Ahab. Ahab is the ancestor, the father of the issues at hand within the body. You could say that Ahab is the issue stirring up trouble within the body. Obadiah isn't sold on going to tell Ahab that Elijah is present. Why is the Elijah Healing process picking on Obadiah? The verse states: "What have I sinned, that you would deliver your servant into the hand of Ahab, to slay me?" Appears Obadiah is playing the role of healthy cells.

Obadiah has followed the Laws of the Universe throughout his life. Notice the reference to sin and how the Universal Law lifestyle which Obadiah follows is hindered by the actions of ancestors who didn't follow the Laws. Processes in the body with respect to the Elijah Healing plasma cycle become hindered or stop working and the entire body fills up with contaminated fluid or muddy water. When the contaminated cells outnumber the healthy cells, there's trouble brewing!

Obadiah informs Elijah of the previous acts Ahab has taken involving nations and kingdoms. Ahab has been on the lookout for Elijah for some time. This situation presents a picture of the fact that ancestor imprints have been passing through generations for quite some time because the Elijah Healing has not been in action. The Elijah Healing process was thrown out many years ago and the Ahab ancestor genetics keep circling around one generation after another. Another contributor to the disappearance of the Elijah Healing is the heavens themselves shifted and the necessary cosmic signals the body needs to move through the cleansing process did not exist. I have good news! The heavens are making a shift back into their intended and beneficial positions, so the human body has the capability of receiving the necessary signals. Now, with the unveiling of ancient wisdom through proper interpretation, the Elijah Healing is making its comeback!

The cleansing service that the body was designed to have has shut down in every nation. There are numerous therapies and treatments that attempt to correct the malfunction of the body, yet all remain unsuccessful at resolving the root genetic issues. While the oath mentioned in these verses may not be known to us today, the secondary definition of an oath is: a coarse or blasphemous word or phrase used to express anger or other strong emotion. Given this, could every curse word that is spoken resurrect an ancient oath and ignite the fire of the original oath imposed? Every nation has been influenced by this oath and resulting disruption in the natural cleansing process. Life and death are in the power of the tongue according to Proverbs 18:21. There is not one people group that has escaped the curse of contaminated plasma. Herein is good reason that our yes should remain yes and our no should be no, without expanding the statement with any other words.

The body responds to the commands it is given through genetic inheritance. The Spirit Energy (chemical elements) and cosmic signals control whether the cleansing process will take place or not. The process can be present or easily swept away. When the genetic inheritances, good or bad, cannot locate the Elijah Healing that keeps the cleaning service running properly, the entire cleansing process of the body is at a minimum slowed down, if not entirely shut down. Toxic water/plasma in the body is a root of soul death and physical decay. Fresh clean water is a must for the body to have the ability to remove toxic debris, and I am not referring to drinking a glass of water. The body was designed to hydrate itself when all meridians are functioning properly and the necessary chemical elements which I call Heavenly Gases, are in place. It is one thing to "be called home/heaven" and it is another to die. The reference to youth tells me a child would receive the necessary Elijah components naturally, but once the age of "youth" is established, the burden of maintaining the health of the meridians and balance of Heavenly Gases becomes an individual responsibility.

The lack of interaction with nighttime cosmic activity eliminates aspects that are described as prophets. My studies and observations today have brought a conclusion that nighttime cosmic activity initiates through the female, thus the reference to the terms union and husband. The female then processes the cosmic delivery received and at the appropriate time delivers a version of the cosmic product to the male. The process can be compared to conception (from the cosmos), pregnancy and birth, delivering an heir/child to the male bloodline. This receiving and distribution has nothing to do with physical intimate activity. This transfer is done on a cellular level.

A supernatural intervention through Obadiah is at work in these verses. A cave represents being removed from the mainstream of life; isolated from the crowd; limited interaction. For the body to receive the necessary Heavenly Gases and put them to use, physical activity must be limited. The more active you are, the more the gases will evaporate. The ancient genetics within must be guarded!

When the Heavenly Gases are not in place, the genetic imprints from ancestors or from a lifestyle that afflicts the blood (alcoholism, smoking, viruses or bacteria that are not properly addressed, etc.), result in situations that will deliver you to the cemetery prematurely.

Verses 15-18: The time has come for the Elijah Healing to meet the genetic imprints. Preparations for this has been followed and completed and now the next step comes into play. Elijah Healing is going to come face-to-face with the genetics inherited from ancestors.

Ahab now accuses Elijah of being the troublemaker for Israel. Elijah has a solid comeback to this accusation stating how it is the Ahab (ancestors) who failed to follow the Commands of the Lord that are causing the health problems. Instead, the Israelites chose to follow the other gods of the world (medical system, education system, etc.), called the Baalim. Today, Baalim will appear in the form of medical and dental industries, rules dealt out by religions, or government guidelines for education. The systems and industries syndrome in the world today. There are many Baalim that fall under the category of being in opposition to the Commands that produce good health and longevity.

During the Elijah Healing, it will seem as though the Elijah Healing process is producing numerous physical discomforts, but on the contrary, it is the inherited imprints when confronted with the Elijah Healing that break out into chaos. I experienced debilitating fatigue, blisters in my mouth, a rash around the base of my nose and outer edges of my mouth that felt like a sunburn. To this symptom I give credit to the multiple ancestors who had years of a cigarette smoking habit! All sorts of red bumps and lumps appeared on my skin, and my hair began falling out. I passed out twice, both times resulting in a concussion that put me in bed for multiple days. My blood sugar plummeted, and my body had bouts of electrical shocking sensations in various places. I will repeat again, this process of eliminating the genetic imprints is not easy, nor is it comfortable. Ladies, gentlemen, youth and elderly, the Baalim is every form of physical treatment or therapy that lies outside the confines of the Elijah Healing and connection to cosmic activity. The body must be allowed to process and eliminate the genetic activity that is wreaking havoc on the body. All forms of interruption to that process only hinder the intended goal. The only intervention I had was to calm episodes of Iritis that progressed to the point I lost the vision in my left eye for approximately six weeks. Iritis is very painful so once I reached the point of unbearable pain, I took Ibuprofen and consulted an optometrist who provided me with a steroid to relieve the pressure on the iris. The least interference you subject your body to during the Elijah Healing, the better the process will work. Given this, there may be times a person must seek medical intervention to avoid premature death or disability. If a person has a broken leg, they need to seek medical attention. If a person is having a heart attack, they need to seek medical attention. The point is, be selective on what needs medical intervention and what can be tolerated. Any form of medical treatment will cause a stall-out in the Elijah Healing process. It is valuable and can be lifesaving to become educated in the process the body goes through to eliminate toxic cells. Most important is positioning yourself so the body can shed the toxic cells. This shedding happens during the season of Fall (Autumn).

<u>Verses 19-24</u>: Israel gets called up to Mount Carmel (what comes through from seed) along with the Baal and Asherah who are in unison with Jezebel (no husband; having no honor; not honoring God's Commands/Laws).

Israel is reference to a people group that belong to "God" yet have stepped away from the Commands (Laws of the Universe) for healthy living. This group has a unique quality in their DNA that will initiate the Elijah Healing in their body. Mount Carmel is a reference to garden or vineyard. A garden is the place of the seed (DNA). A vineyard is reflective of a vine, being connected to Jesus who is the vine, and we who live like Jesus did are the branches. (John 15:5). Living like Jesus does not equate to being a good person. Living like Jesus is walking through the steps His life shows us through isolation, hardships, rejection, torture, and so forth. With all this comes clean blood!

Elijah Healing confronts the contaminated DNA seed with: verse 21, "How long will you dance between two opinions?" Elijah is pointing out the fact that you cannot have two masters. Either the Commands/Laws are your master or worldly living is your master. Following the Commands will result in a peaceful departure from the earth and worldly living will result in some form of disastrous, costly or painful departure. Hopefully not all three. Either you trust in God with the Elijah Healing, or you trust in the other forms of medical treatments and therapies. There is no mixing the two that will result in a pleasant outcome. Trust God or trust man is the choice.

Now Elijah is giving instruction for putting the bull to the fire. A bull represents DNA, seed, sperm. Notice the instruction includes Baals bull being cut in pieces. Could the cutting of the bull represent a form of DNA damage, fragmented. This sounds like destruction of the "seed" but is there something specific about the DNA that becomes damaged beyond repair? Yet, Elijah's bull remains in one piece, no interruption or damage to the seed/DNA. There are numerous (450 recognized in these verses) health related reports that are produced by the Baals. The Elijah Healing works alone. No need for manmade potions, lotions or outsider assistance. Wood represents portions of the family tree.

Next, the fire is called down. Fire is a form of destruction, to return something to ash, to eliminate. Fire can be thought of as a way to do a thorough cleansing, taking things down to the core.

<u>Verses 25-29</u>: Bulls are now prepared, and the prophets of Baal begin to call on their gods. What are some of the gods they might call on? Surgeries, prescription drugs, vaccinations or immunizations, etc. The Baals try different forms of shouting and leaping but their gods did not respond. It appears remedies of the medical industry are not working. Elijah takes action and at noon begins to make fun of their attempts that are producing no response.

Noon is an indication of a change in the measure of cosmic activity (culmination)or chemical elements in the environment that happens at that specific time. Talking, relieving himself, being on a journey and sleeping all refer to the physical, something that is done in the material world. Keep in mind these four physical activities talking, relieving yourself/using the bathroom, a journey or any form of travel which includes by foot or by vehicle, exposure to the sun, and sleep, as we move along.

In verse 28, the prophets certainly have an influence on the blood. The use of knives and lancets (or spears) would be a reference to surgeries, cutting someone open. For blood to gush out of a cut is not a small one but indicates the cut is more along the lines of opening someone up.

An act of prophesying took place "until the time of the offering of the afternoon sacrifice." The frame of time referenced is equivalent to standard office hours. No fire comes to the bull (seed) and the sacrifice (disruptive symptoms) is not consumed. Fire is reference to an element that consumes through a fuel, in this case internal gases.

The proper combination and balance of Heavenly Gases will cause a form of internal fire that will consume seed/DNA imprints. Let's see what happens when Elijah calls on God.

<u>Verses 30-35</u>: *The altar (an elevated or high structure; location where sacrifices took place) inside the body has become broken. The altar represents the place where contamination is taken away, things are burned up and removed. When the Elijah Healing is in place, the process described as animal sacrifice is a depiction of how the Elijah Healing destroys the various contaminations that have come into the body that will ultimately destroy the seed/DNA if not addressed. This is not a reference to a daily dose of car exhaust or cleansing solutions. This is speaking of contaminated cells, the DNA that becomes afflicted. The word altar could be replaced with alterations. Such as alterations in the seed/DNA will be burned up with internal fire when the Elijah Healing is applied.*

The broken altar describes a result of the oath spoken that interrupted the production of clean water inside the body causing muddy water to take over. Refer to verses 7-14 of Chapter 18. An altar is an elevated status (or raised, as in superior) inside the body where the fire (gases) performs their partnership duties while moving along with the plasma (water).

Next, Elijah takes 12 stones that represent the 12 sons of Jacob, and the Lord gave utterance to Elijah who states, "Israel will be your name." Twelve stones are in the Ephod. The stones of the Ephod should be used during the Elijah Healing. The stones can be worn or simply carried in a pocket. The stones attract the gases necessary for the internal fire. This verse also indicates the Elijah Healing is for those who belong to the people group discussed above. I call this people group Hebrews versus Jews simply to avoid the confusion with a religious practice. Today, the term Hebrew is not limited to persons born in Israel, or who has ancestral roots in or from Israel.

The details of a sacrifice are now described, giving rise to the notion that descendants of any of the 12 sons of Jacob will and can be used as a form of sacrifice "to the Lord." Water becomes a component in this detailed description. Again, in many verses, the water reference is used for representation of the plasma in the blood. Measurements of seed can indicate the DNA from mom and the DNA from dad. There is a specific measure of water the body will produce to accompany the process of elimination of genetic imprints. This cycle of events is done three times and is time consuming. The body goes through natural cycles, and those cycles can take days, weeks, months or years.

Verses 36-46: Notice the time of "afternoon" is given. Something specific with respect to the process of the Elijah Healing is taking place after the sun has reached its peak of the day. The verses go on to state, "let it be known this day that You are God in Israel." I bring your attention to the word "in." Replace the word "in" with "within," meaning internal, not amongst as "in" would indicate. Being a servant is a strong indication that there is certain work being done by those who fall under the description of Israel (or Israelite) that is for the "Lord." This is where the photosynthesis-like activity comes in. It is as though the human body transforms magnetic pulses or chemical elements that are present in the earth. An action that reconstructs them or maybe even causes a change in negative/positive ions. Interesting nonetheless and would make for a good movie.

We must shed a different light upon the word "Lord." The word "Lord" supports a meaning of "that which has authority over you" or "being of high rank." It will cause great confusion to place upon the word "Lord" the imagery of the physical manifestation of who we know as "Jesus." Lord, in these verses, is not a reference to a person but a condition or influence present in the air (chemical elements) that surrounds us. History also reveals the title of Lord was given to those who were landowners.

Elijah mentions the act of "turning the heart," which is a strong indicator that the Elijah Healing process being described has a great influence on the physical heart muscle. This is not an emotional trip. It is an adventure of walking through ancestral markers (genetically) and eliminating them through the power of certain acts that must take place in alignment with the planets that will bring about a properly functioning physical heart muscle. There is a joint effort taking place between God (Heavenly Gases in the body) and the Elijah Healing. Elijah provides a service to give God the resources necessary to address the issues at hand. The reference to heart indicates a cardiac reset takes place.

Notice "fire of the Lord." Again this is reference to specific measure and combination of chemical elements I call Heavenly Gases. The gases come together and remove the damaged fragments of the family tree that includes the Israelites and all the way back to the dust that Adam was formed from. In other words, all the way to the origins. The gases move the water in the body to wash the debris out of the body. Notice how Elijah first summoned the orchestration of the bull as a sacrifice that needed fire and in this verse the sacrifice is already burnt before the fire falls. This tells me the work of the Elijah Healing sweeps the debris into one location so the Heavenly Gases can move through and activate the final cleansing process.

Elijah gives the instruction to, "Catch the prophets of Baal!" The prophets of Baal are gathered up, taken to Elijah and what takes place? The Elijah Healing eliminates them. Prophets of Baal are the medical or dental diagnosis or treatments received by a person or their ancestors, or both, that cause contamination to take over cells. The work of the plasma is going to remove all contamination the body has received through prescription drugs, treatments, surgeries or radiation, and so forth.

Sounds like the influence from treatments and therapies many have come to use and rely on are going to be eliminated. It is my hope that this would be in response to people learning how to properly apply the Elijah Healing. Once the initial Elijah Healing process is complete, maintenance (of the plasma) is a breeze.

When the prophets (the genetic soundbites that dictate your health and future) are eliminated, it swings the door open for the healthy genetics from ancestors to be called forth. Clean blood and plasma mean healthy cells from ancestors have room to grow, to multiply. The Law of Attraction comes into play. Live according to the Commands and the cells (good genetics) from ancestors who lived according to the Commands will come forth. Here is where I think of the 14 generations listed in Matthew, Chapter 1. Those 14 generations are listed for a reason other than just to show us who begat whom. They are listed to tell us that our blood can carry genes of ancestors 14 generations back.

Ahab takes off to find a snack while Elijah goes for a hike up to the top of Mount Carmel. Elijah appears to have an expectation of change, a shift in the atmosphere. The reference to "a man's hand" is an indication of works or application of something of man's doing, not God's doing. To "go back" is a reference to generational lines. Seven generations of toxic imprints caused by the work of man's hand. A hand is representative of a trade or skill, and most importantly, how you handle business or personal affairs. When a person consults a business or professional for a diagnosis or other conclusive report, there is a money exchange. You pay for the services requested and that transaction makes a type of bond between you and the business or professional consulted. If that business or professional has any connection to over-charging for the services rendered, dishonesty, forms of service that may involve a type of trickery, is unfair and so forth, the connection made allows a measure of the conduct to attach to the consultee's life. In other words, the consequences of thievery, dishonesty, trickery, robbery, unfair dealings, dishonest trade, and the like, will trickle down a generational line to the seventh generation when a form of agreement has been made. What you are joined or connected to will attract an element of same in a like-manner to you. Good or bad. Again, the Law of Attraction comes into play. Those who have built empires on dishonest acts have paved the road for their descendants to pay a big price, and this dishonesty attaches to those who form an agreement or exchange with them/it. God does not take criminal acts lightly. Jude 1:14 describes how every seventh generation will endure the consequences for the previous six generations of sins. Ouch!

Ahab is given the instruction to "harness his chariot." Chariots have a connection to the wheels/chakras that run along the center of the body. In Traditional Chinese Medicine acupuncture, chariots are the jaws. Rain is the subject now and it becomes voluminous. Ahab prepares the chariot and goes to Jezreel. Looking at the definition of Jezreel we discover: Seed, offspring, sowing, seat of strength, scatter; he will be sown of God are components at play. Seed is DNA or cells, add in "sown of God" and we have a measure of the cells in the body that contain an element of God, something that was planted or placed by God's handiwork. As the chapters move forward, remember the references here to jaw and rain which is discussed in detail in Chapter 9.

The transition footrace is on. The Elijah Healing hops to it and scurries to Jezreel (the seed/cells placed in the body by God) in front of Ahab (ancestors who followed the ways of the world).

The ancestorial genetics that are healthy and a benefit will escape the cleansing waters that wash through to clear out the toxic debris. The Elijah Healing process secures the God-enhanced cells/DNA. The next phase is for the cells/DNA to become built with Heavenly Gases.

CHAPTER 3
1 KINGS, CHAPTER 19

THE THREAT OF DEATH

<u>Verses 1-10</u>: The report of Elijah slaying the prophets reaches the ears of Jezebel through the mouth of Ahab. Prophets are persons who deliver the messages authored by the divine or supernatural figures. Prophets are also the genetic soundbites that dictate your health situations, present and future. It appears that there is a form of unpleasant messages coming through 'Ahab ancestors' and any message from an ancestor would mean the messages are recorded in the blood, DNA, genetics. Jezebel is not happy about Elijah's actions and gives an oath: "So let the gods do to me (Jezebel) and more also, if I do not make your life like the life of one of them by tomorrow about this time." Sounds like Jezebel is a real threat to the Elijah Healing. Let's look back and see what Jezebel means again. Jezebel is the "no Husband" syndrome. Husband is a word of choice used in the bible to direct attention to a cosmic activity that involves the moon and its influence on the physical body. When a person does not know how to position themselves for receiving the moon influence, the Elijah Healing is jeopardized. It is a benefit to know how to dance with the moon, so to speak.

The Elijah Healing escapes for its well-being and goes to Beer-Sheba, the well (deep or down under) of oath (promise). A promise that exists on the interior of the body. This promise has a unique connection to

Judah. The Elijah Healing leaves its co-worker(s) in Beer-Sheba and continues its journey to the wilderness where resting under a juniper tree is in order. The reference to juniper tree could indicate there is a measure of support to the healing process through the means of an essential oil of juniper. Juniper and Balsam tree oils are beneficial June-August, currently the summer months. Elijah is tired, ready to give up. It has been taxing on Elijah to go through the healing process required to protect the seed/DNA.

Now we have a situation where ancestor(s) made an oath that has now trickled down to the seventh generation. It is a situation where the oath and its consequences remain alive in all seasons, represented by the hardy juniper tree, an evergreen. These generational oaths can create situations where you feel hopeless because everything you do seems to not work well for you, indicated by Elijah's desire to die, yet there are situations where an oath of benefit can be at play. God made a promise to His people, a beneficial oath. It is important to note here that an oath is also a swearing, whether a formal swearing as in a courtroom or the use of general verbal swearing as in cuss words. Using swear words will not only make their way back to you but will follow the generational lines and create unpleasant situations for descendants. Elijah is fed up with dealing with the consequences, or you could say curse(s), left behind by the ancestors. Jezebel threatening to track Elijah down is this ever-haunting feeling that something is going to take your life. You can clean up genetic imprints from ancestor eating habits, clothing choices and such but overcoming a generational oath that creates a curse is much more challenging. Looking back over the prior six and seven generations to discover what may have been said can be a challenge. Most often a person has no idea what their ancestors that far back took part in. One oath issue I have come across is military oaths. Any oath will throw some form of curse into the generations. Our yes should be yes, and no should be no. Being dedicated to something is one thing but giving an oath binds the bloodline to the oath given.

The Elijah Healing must have the nourishment that comes from fresh baked tortillas. I say tortillas because the bread must be free of any form of leavening. Leavenings create gases in the body, and those gases need to be avoided for the Elijah Healing process to perform its duties. Do not drink water. The bible references water but too much water in the body causes the gases that are created by the fresh bread to be extinguished. Drink Concord Grape juice. It contains chromium that the body needs during the healing process. The intake of bread and juice must be done after sunset. I continue to eat a fresh tortilla and drink Concord Grape juice each evening as maintenance. I want no toxic disruption to take up residence in my blood.

The Elijah Healing process takes time and a lot of energy. There will be times when you may feel like giving up, hiding in a cave like Elijah did. It can become discouraging simply because the general population has no idea what is taking place in their body on a cellular level. No one can relate to what you are going through. You feel as though you are walking through a challenging journey with no visible results to prove that it is working. My best advice is, hang in there! The results come but it can take weeks, months and even years for visible evidence to be present. Elijah describes the magnitude of the mess he has worked at cleaning up: "I have been very zealous for the Lord God of Hosts for the children of Israel have forsaken Your covenant, thrown down Your altars, and slain Your prophets with the sword. And only I am left, and they seek my life to take it away." The ability to receive the opportunity to go through an Elijah Healing process can be snuffed out. "God's prophets" references the genetics within a person that are from ancestors who followed the Laws. When those genes are destroyed, there is no chance of overcoming the disease sentence placed upon you.

<u>Verses 11-16:</u> describe various physical symptoms, relating them to weather occurrences. ... *a great and strong wind tore the mountains and broke the rocks in pieces before the Lord, but the Lord was not in the wind. And after the wind an earthquake, but the Lord was not in the earthquake. And after the earthquake a fire, but the Lord was not in the fire. And after the fire a still small voice.* Notice the Lord was not involved in these various disturbing situations? The finger of blame points to the actions of ancestors that planted the seeds for varying forms of destruction.

Elijah comes out of his cave experience and begins to appoint ruling powers, noted as kings, to oversee various areas. These instructions are given to Elijah: He is to return to the wilderness of Damascus (well-watered place; hydrated), cause Hazael (window, to see or experience) to be king over Syria (Straight or upright; decisive progression, to make things right; a walk or a going; happiness; tree (family tree)); to anoint Jehu (Wailing, muffled groaning, labored utterance), the son of Nimshi (Rescued from danger), king over Israel. And anoint Elisha (Salvation through/by God), the son of Shafat (To judge, governor; a ruling in a penal sense; ordinance, custom or manner) from Abel Meholah (meadow or stream + to dance or whirl) to be prophet in his place. Whew! That was a mouthful. It appears the Elijah Healing process is nearing its completion and specific energetic shifts or powers are now in position. Israel, the tribal group that strayed from the Laws put in place by God, are rescued from the dangers of the loss of their soul life. The beneficial ancestor genetics are resurrected and do their dance, producing health for the body. We could call this: Resurrecting the dead! (Revelation 20:5-6)

<u>Verses 17-21</u>: *Jehu will slay the one who escapes the sword of Hazael and Elisha will slay the one who escapes from the sword of Jehu.*

The references to "one" is genetic imprints. If you don't have a physical reaction during the Elijah Healing process, you will have a time of grieving, moaning or challenged utterance. These can all be signs of the genetic contamination making its way out of the body.

Seven thousand remain in Israel, a small fraction of today's population, that have not bowed the knees to Baal and not elevated reports thereof. There are a few good DNA strands in the mix that have not been contaminated by some form of worldly contamination.

Elisha comes on the scene noting a shift. Elisha is the offspring of Shafat and Shafat means to judge, governor; a ruling in a penal sense; ordinance, custom or manner. Shafat's act of plowing with 12 yoke of oxen gives us a message of working the field, hard work; an act or issue that is tied around the neck usually with little or no escape. Oxen work the soil, and the physical body is constructed from the "dust of the ground" (Genesis 2:7). What is a field? Field is the expanse where energy exists that has a connection to the physical body, the soil. A field can also represent a space owned and tended to by a specific group of people or a person. The verse states Shafat was with the "twelfth." This sounds a little random. Shafat is working a field and all of the sudden the focus shifts to the "twelfth." Twelfth son of the twelve tribes is Benjamin – strength that comes from being classified as a "Son." The Elijah Healing has advanced to the point of producing "sonship" that is in a position of strength (right hand). What does the tribe of Benjamin have to do with these events? Elisha (salvation) is a member of the tribe of Benjamin. I will propose that the actual descendants of the tribe of Benjamin are (or should have been) the main players in the work of the field, the energy field. The tribe of Benjamin dropped the ball, and salvation was no longer available in a health sense. Because of the lack of knowledge, and a dash of being "set in their ways," this ball that brings life will be placed in reliable hands. A different tribal group will begin the work that maintains a balance in the electro-magnetic field that surrounds us and which brings help with respect to the cyclical activity necessary for keeping the body healthy. People are responsible for following the Laws of the Universe (for their own salvation, so to speak) to receive this assistance that comes through cellular signaling. It would be like this: I could help you on a cellular level to overcome a temporary affliction like the flu, but you are personally responsible for the day-to-day requirements that involve food, clothing choices, sleep, etc. More on this subject will come forth in future publications.

The Elijah Healing becomes Elisha (salvation, which means rescue). The Elijah Healing job duties have now produced rescue from the genetic imprints. Elisha takes steps to depart from family, specifically his parents. In this situation, the story is speaking of the separation from contaminated DNA that comes through the parents. Elisha plays the role of the separation from the genetic imprints that pass through the parents DNA so Elisha (as salvation) can more easily follow in the footsteps of Elijah (the Elijah Healing) by bringing the necessary healing that keeps the physical body healthy.

CHAPTER 4
1 KINGS, CHAPTER 20

WHAT'S ALL THE NOISE ABOUT?

<u>Verses 1-6</u>: Ben-Hadad (noise or commotion) steps into the picture and gathers his army. There are thirty-two ruling powers (kings are what rule over people and horses are power) that use the jaw/mouth. Chariots are instruments that carry you away or take you for a ride, just as the words spoken or food eaten through the jaw/mouth can take you for a ride in health or thoughts. Sometimes going for a ride is not such a good idea. The jaw would be specific to chewing and chewing is an act of preparing something to be ingested.

Feuds arise and war breaks out. Then Ahab receives a message that he will be stripped of all his valuables. Gold, silver, wives and children. These ancestor issues have become a real mess. The wealth, spouse and children, will all be influenced by what your body is exposed to. The influence is not just to your body but to the cells that signal to those who carry genes much like yours. Ben-Hadad sent the command claiming the right to possess valuables. King Ahab bows to the command and turns over the valuables to the noise makers. What is this saying? Excess exposure to noise can result in chaos inside the body. The nervous system will respond to the noise that has been recorded in the cells. The cell begins to play the disco (noise or commotion) recording, and the nervous system responds. The body and a person's brain function will eventually follow in the footsteps of its master. To expose the body to even the voice of a teacher (education or religion) who is not in complete alignment with what God commands can be deadly for the teacher, the student and their families. Noise appears to have become a commander. This is a good place to insert Jeremiah 6:14 and 8:11 (HCS): They have treated superficially the brokenness of My dear people, claiming, 'Peace, peace,' when there is no peace. The chaotic cells need peace!

Many times, valuables are not tangible items but things such as health, or favor with God. Taking a little different view on valuables being turned over to a noise making component (Ben-Hadad), the brain cells suffer greatly when it is subjected to loud or continual forms of noise. Noise can be found in many forms and places. Forms of noise that can cause the greatest damage comes from microphones and speakers that amplify sound, machinery, large crowds, concerts and musical instruments in general.

<u>Verses 7-14:</u> continue to describe the demise that comes with submission to noise in its various forms. Once you submit, if you decide to depart from the authority given, you will have a spiritual fight on your hands. The mind becomes addicted to what it has been fed and the body will resist any change implemented to erase the disruptive recordings. Easily said, the devil does not willingly depart from territory he was once given. In time, God will send rescue.

<u>Verses 15-25</u>: Princes are powers of or within the air, the atmosphere. There is mention of noon time and a chemical reaction described as drunk. An influence found in the blood. A form of being inebriated comes with sabotaging the brain with noise: "If they march out in peace, take them alive and if they have marched out for battle, take them alive." Any way you slice it, your life is at risk.

Many things can take place at noon. People take their lunch break from work at or near noon; many church services dismiss around noon. With the symbol of Ben-Hadad being commotion and noise, I will again direct your attention to church services, restaurants where noise abounds, sporting events that are accompanied by loudspeakers and music. This is not the first time I have written about the dangers of being inside the walls of a church building, restaurant or sports complex while music and voices are pushed through high-definition speaker systems. This noise causes gases in the atmosphere to dissolve or change, and the collection of altered gases will cause an influence in the blood. This is the picture being set forth through the character of Ben-Hadad, drunk, and the death sentence issued. One can conclude that any form of activity, outside of a quiet meditation during the hour of noon to 1:00 p.m., causes a health risk to the body, particularly the blood. (Psalm 46:10; Matthew 26:40; 1 Corinthians 14:15)

There is mention of a seasonal change connected to when powers will come against a person yet again. Some translations list this seasonal change as Spring, some say Fall and some say at the "return of the year." I'll leave this debate for a later date but will point out that this is the type of thing that happens when there are multiple "new year" markers and multiple theologians with their hand in the pot of translations and interpretations. A "new year" can reflect the beginning of a new cycle. Whatever the correct marker(s) is, it brings another round of attack. Syria represents something from long ago. There is no clear definition for the word Syria other than the region. This issue from long ago is going to "come up against you" in the form of ups and downs in your health. Any way you look at it, the body will shift to a new phase at a seasonal marker.

<u>Verses 26-34</u>: Now the story has come to the "turn of the year" when this issue from long ago (Syria) comes alive. Aphek (confinement of a water passage) appears to be an issue in those with Hebrew blood. Acts of attempting to get the location, and magnitude of the war that is set to breakout begin. For seven days the debate continues. Is this notation of seven days a reference to the seven years it takes to complete the Elijah Healing process? Or, the necessity of there being seven days to work through a particular cycle inside the body?

There's a shift in which powers are at play now as stated, "... we have heard that the kings of the House of Israel are kings of lovingkindness." Ahab then acknowledges that Ben-Hadad is a blood relative of his, one of the same root bloodlines. Ahab (ancestor genes) and Ben-Hadad (commotion, noise) meet, and an agreement is made that the things the ancestors destroyed should be replaced. Inherited noise imprints are at play and must be replaced. Cooperation at last!

<u>Verses 35-43</u>: An interesting description is held within these verses regarding what can come upon the physical body when the Commands (when to eat, what to eat, etc.) are not followed. The attack to the body is compared to that of a lion. The survival rate from an attack of a lion is quite slim. Then again, some people will survive the physical attacks when they come at them with what is compared to being struck by another human. Maybe a cut here and there and some bumps and bruising are had. Is this description of attacks indicative of the various levels of physical symptoms or outbreaks a person might experience during their Elijah Healing? Some people will survive the attacks, and some will not. Horrible thought but true, nonetheless.

To expand on the previous paragraph, walk with me through a series of thoughts. Thinking of Judah, the tribe specifically set out in Scripture as having strayed (from the Laws and Commands). Judah is also connected to the "lion of the tribe of Judah" (the bloodline of Jesus). Could this equate to the Judah tribe members having a larger responsibility than others when it comes to the Elijah Healing? A form of taking on more of the load of "sin" (genetic imprints) than the remainder of the descendants of Jacob? Possibly a situation where a Judah descendant can help someone of another tribe eliminate the contaminated signals coming from the genetic imprints they have? Does the phrase "cleansing the sins of many" ring any bells? (Hebrews 9:28) Note that the verse itself is located in the book of Hebrews.

Consider the story of Ruth and Boaz. Boaz was a member of the Judah descendants. Ruth Chapter 3, verses 12-13 states: Yes, it is true that I (Boaz) am a family redeemer, but there is a redeemer closer than I am. Stay here tonight and in the morning if he wants to redeem you, that's good. Let him redeem you. But if he doesn't want to redeem you, as the Lord lives, I will. Now lie down until morning. (HCS) I want to point out a few key things in these verses. First, Ruth was a Moabite, coming from the bloodline of Lot and his son Moab who was born out of incest, but married into the Judah tribe. A sort of adoption took place that grafted Ruth into the Judah bloodline. Second, notice how Ruth is told to "lie down until morning." This indicates there is an activity that takes place during the nighttime hours that can redeem you but if for some reason it does not, a family member can. The "redeemer" closer to Ruth than Boaz is the electro-magnetic activity of the cosmos and/or chemical elements produced thereof (sometimes referred to as "God"). Interesting thoughts for sure. It all sounds like a far-stretch now but knowing how cell signals communicate and receive signals (vibrations) from other objects, I would say there is more truth in this thought pattern than one would want to believe.

There are people assigned to receive messages from God, from the cosmos. Not everyone receives these types of messages. The next few verses tell us that a prophet (person with the message) paused and waited for the correct power (king) but was not recognized by the power that would approach. Ashes represent having been through the fire, the situations that burn away that which is harmful, no longer valuable or useful. So, this prophet tells the story of how a person with the title of servant, delivered a physical being to him. A servant is someone who performs work in the realm of balancing magnetics or identifying and balancing an electrical charge that has become harmful. This is sometimes called energy work. The servant had a dangerous situation on his hands (battle) and needed the power that <u>resides within a prophet</u> to protect the physical body or physical aspects of the servant. While the servant is doing his job energetically, he needs support or direction through someone who has a connection to the information from above – God's messages, the application and function of the Laws of the Universe. In the previous chapters I describe a prophet as being the ancestor genetics, often several generations back, that are healthy genes from the ones who followed the Laws. Are there a percentage of people who have "servant genetics" in their blood? Is it possible that people with prophet genes help those with servant genes?

In the physical sense, the job of the prophet is no easy one. A prophet may be held accountable for someone's life if the prophet does not deliver the proper message(s) and the servant incurs great harm or death (Deuteronomny 18:18-22). Being a prophet carries a serious job description and should not be taken lightly. Not everyone can be a prophet, and certainly not everyone can become a prophet by *attending a class. No matter who their earthly teacher is. God appoints prophets, not mankind, which tells me the title of prophet comes through the genetics. Once a message from a true prophet is delivered to you, the weight lies in your hands as to how you respond to the message and any consequences thereof are now yours.*

CHAPTER 5
1 KINGS, CHAPTER 21

THE VINEYARD TOO?

<u>Verses 1-4</u>: In this chapter Ahab's interest becomes directed at Naboth's vineyard. Ahab attempts to cut a deal with Naboth by offering an equal parcel of land or silver for the vineyard. Naboth means to bear fruit, a sprout or fertility. It appears Naboth is fertile with something important. Jezreel means seed, offspring, sowing, seat of strength, scatter; he will be sown of God. There is something special about Naboth's DNA and Ahab must be apprised of the fact that Naboth has the DNA code that connects him to the heavens, the cosmos. Naboth is a part of the all-important "vine."

Naboth rejects Ahab's offers stating: "I will never give my fathers' (ancestors) inheritance to you." It sounds like the healthy genetics produced through ancestors who followed the Laws is safe from any influence the contaminated genes (Ahab) carry. This is really good news!

<u>Verses 5-6</u>: Jezebel steps on the scene and inquires of Ahab why he is downtrodden. Ahab, what's up? Ahab shares with Jezebel the conversation he had with Naboth.

<u>Verses 7-14</u>: Jezebel pulls out the royal power card and tells Ahab she will deal with Naboth. Jezebel writes a letter and forges

Ahab's name upon it. First boo-boo, forgery is a no-no! The letters instructed elders and nobles to proclaim a fast, with Naboth positioned at the head of the table. Fasting for a person who is part of the "vine" can be deadly. Such fasting, being complete removal of all food, is considered blasphemy to God and any ruling powers (healthy cells) within the body. Jezebel instructs that Naboth's position was to be between two wicked men who would claim Naboth had blasphemed God and the king. Jezebel is wicked in her scheme to gain possession of the vineyard. Lying is a cousin of forgery. Jezebel is on a role here. She wanted Naboth out the way. For Jezebel to proclaim a fast there is an element of demise attached to it.

A note of caution should be placed on the definition we have for fasting today. Elimination of all food and drink for lengthy periods can damage healthy cells. There is a risk of eliminating the very genetics that will pull you through the Elijah Healing process! This is evident through the reference to Naboth being accused of blasphemy. So, what is really happening here in this scene? Jezebel's name means no husband. There is an activity initiated by the cosmos that attracts to people with a specific DNA code in their blood. Naboth, one who is of the vine, had that DNA code, the healthy genes. To be without the cosmic activity labeled as "husband" causes the DNA code to be removed, a loss of the connection to the vineyard. Ahab, as king, represents the power that came against God's people who were connected to the vine and had the connection with cosmic activity, to lose their DNA code. I can only speculate here but I would say the specific DNA code is received during development of the fetus in the womb. It would be initiated by cosmic activity such as a specific moon phase or maybe an eclipse or some form of specific event of the heavens.

<u>Verses 15-16</u>: With Naboth out of the way, Ahab jumps at the chance to take possession of the vineyard. When the Naboth (the origins of good genetics) are depleted, the contaminated genes take over. This is troubling, especially given that we currently have no way of knowing what percentage of "good" genes we have nor how fast, or by what all various means they can be eliminated. Sounds like a situation where we are walking around in the dark. Is this where "walk by faith and not by sight" comes in?

<u>Verses 17-26</u>: Elijah has connections with God messages and hears of the events that took place between Ahab (contaminated ancestor genes), Jezebel (no connection to the cosmic activity) and Naboth (origins of good genetics). Elijah makes his way to Ahab's castle and tells Ahab he is aware of the situation involving the vineyard. Elijah has a specific message for Ahab: "In the place where dogs licked the blood of Naboth, dogs will lick your blood." This is a rather strange statement. Let's unravel what it means. Dog is the term used to describe people who follow the commands of mankind, they travel in packs (groups) and often eat anything put in front of them. The blood is obviously influenced, meaning consumed, by the dog. The Elijah Healing is going to eliminate the Ahab contaminated cells in the same manner Naboth was eliminated.

This could lead us to a conclusion that a group of people were involved in the removal of the practices and teachings on how to join the cosmic husband activity. This in turn influenced the blood to the point it erased the DNA code (good genes). Hmm, there's one of the destructive issues, no cosmic activity or "husband." It also speaks of medical practices that damage the blood on a cellular level. Many reports and statistics that present medical testing as safe do not base their findings on testing done at a cellular level. A "buyer beware" should be attached to those routine exams and scans.

For the removal of instructions and ultimate demise of the cosmic connection, the results pour out upon the group that initiated the plan of destruction. This story holds a good lesson in not altering the ancient instructions given by God thousands of years ago. People have a right to their opinion about a practice or lifestyle but making moves that will ultimately eliminate or alter the original instruction can result in harm beyond our scope of understanding. It is safe to say that the world is currently full of influence that can be deadly to the DNA code, the healthy genetics that come through a cosmic connection. There's no better way to state it than verse 21: This is what the Lord says: "I am about to bring disaster on you and will sweep away your descendants: I will eliminate all of Ahab's males, both slave and free (those who carry contaminated seed and those who do not), in Israel." Jumping to verse 24: "He who belongs to Ahab and dies in the city, the dogs will eat (medical treatments or professional opinions will eat you alive), and he who dies in the field (energy field, relying on manipulation of the electrical function of the body), the birds of the sky will eat."

Why are dogs and birds specifically mentioned? Here's where the wisdom steps into the subject of reincarnation, which is not expanded on in this publication. There are other verses in Scripture that mention the dog and the bird within the same verse as well. Avoiding any argument about whether a soul is bound for reincarnation or not, here is the interpretation of verse 24: If you belong to a "dog" group, meaning those who bow to the Baals by jumping in line for every routine medical exam, vaccination, dental x-rays, and so forth, and shun the activities required to accept the cosmic husband activity, when you die your physical death while in that state of opinion, it is quite possible you will reincarnate as a dog (follower of the world's systems. Example: you return and become a target for medical practices to destroy the good genes, or you become a person who delivers the practices that destroy the good genes) or a bird (you return and become someone who follows the spirit activity, energy related practices that can harm the electrical system in the body). Does a person reincarnate as a literal dog or bird? That question I do not have a solid answer for at this time. Reincarnation lies within the status of the soul (Star Dust) at the time of physical death. Enough on that topic for now.

<u>Verses 27-29</u>: Ahab is distraught about the situation and presents himself in a state of mourning. God is impressed by Ahab's humility and erases the curse spoken to Ahab but keeps it in place for any sons of Ahab. The way you conduct yourself during your life here on earth may not always influence your living situation but will come down the pike to your descendants.

CHAPTER 6
1 KINGS, CHAPTER 22

TAKING POSSESSION OF WHAT IS YOURS

<u>Verses 1-8</u>: For three years life moves along without major interruptions or life-threatening situations. Things become leveled out with respect to health once the daily practices have been put into place. Consequences (aka judgments) arise and Judah's king and Israel's king meet. These two kings represent a unique quality that exists in the Judah bloodline, similar to what is found in Joseph and Bejamin and how they stand out amongst the crowd as compared to the general population of those considered to be of Israelite blood.

The king of Israel said to his servants, "Do you know that Ramot (elevations) in Gilead (perpetual fountain) is ours? The power that is present over the Israelite blood makes an announcement regarding a right to ownership. Something relative to the Elijah Healing and what comes about through that healing has not yet been manifest, in part due to the ones being healed being unaware of what they are entitled to. There is another step that must be taken and that step is described as something that is in the possession of "Syria" (To make things right; straight or upright). To gain possession of this physical aspect, a battle for possession will take place. There will be symptoms, aches, pains, shifts in sleep or alertness. Various things in the physical body will begin to fight for the possession it *is entitled to. This is triggered by cellular activity, and the cycles cells go through. The body will fight to make things correct. It is wise to walk through this process with the direction of the Spirit. Proper meditation is a must and is only productive at specific times of day which is determined solely by the position of the sun. Set your goals, write them on paper and sit quietly during the hour of noon to 1:00 p.m., when the sun is at its peak. As previously mentioned, noise and activity at noon can cause an undesirable influence on the blood. The brain also needs a time to reboot, and noon is the time for that reboot session.*

In the following scene we learn that prophets are consulted about the upcoming battle. It is reported that messages received from prophets can be either uplifting or lack an ability to inspire one about their situation. Whether reports are good or bad should not rest solely upon the shoulders of the prophet. The prophet is simply a medium between a person and the reports received from the records contained in the cosmos. Micaiah (who is like God) the son of Imlah (cycle of harvest, storage and redistribution; wither or weaken; filling of gold with jewels; fullness) appears to have the reputation of delivering bad reports. As you will recall, a prophet is not only a physical person but also the cellular signals that come from ancient healthy genes. Great-great grandpa may be trying to tell you something through those cell signals.

<u>*Verses 9-14*</u>*: Micaiah is summoned to the scene. The kings take their proper position, and the prophesies pour out. The download of messages begins.*

Zedekiah (to be just, righteous) the son of Chenaanah (to synchronize or give up individual leanings to unite as a group; humbled; to bend the knee) steps to the microphone and announces that the Syrians will be consumed during battle and the kings are encouraged to proceed against Syria (family tree) at Ramot Gilead (elevated testimony). Something in the family tree is heating up!

Micaiah had been waiting off in the distance, and he is encouraged to deliver a message in unison with what the others had said. Micaiah reminds the audience that he will report what the Lord says, not necessarily what everyone else has said.

Make note in verse 10 it states that the king of Israel and the king of Judah were clothed in royal attire. This verse is telling us there is royal blood at play in Israelites. I'm not saying in this statement that everyone who qualifies as an Israelite will wear purple and be seated on a literal throne and support a crown on their head. This is speaking of purity in the blood. It also tells us that what is in the blood will reflect to the exterior of the body. Makes sense. The mention of Judah separate from being an Israelite, causes one to wonder if those from the bloodline of Judah have a double portion of the royal blood component, the good genetics. Another line of thought is there are certain standards a royal must live by to maintain the status of being a royal. Jesus, being from the bloodline of Judah, tells us there is something Judah has that the remainder of Israelite tribes do not have. Here's where a laboratory would be beneficial but then how would you know what to test for?

<u>Verses 15-23</u>: The time comes for Micaiah to speak. He encourages the kings to proceed with the battle at Ramot Gilead (elevated + testimony) and having delivered this message he is questioned as to whether he is telling them the truth. Sounds like a typical crowd. They want to hear what they want to hear and when they are told the message they question its validity. One could only imagine how Micaiah would have been frustrated with this crowd by now.

Micaiah delivers the details to the kings: "I saw all Israel scattered upon the hills, like sheep that do not have a shepherd and the Lord said, 'these have no master, let each man return to his house in peace.'" Given this report, it sounds like people these days are scattered in every direction. Some people believe in this, some in that, some seek healthcare with this practice, some with that practice, and so forth. The king of Israel becomes testy and voices his dislike for the comparison of his people to scattered sheep. To avoid being scattered, it sounds like everyone needs to be on the same page!

The plot thickens and plans begin to involve Ahab. Something needs to fall into place so the genetic imprints that are left to descendants can be cleaned up and hauled off. But how is that going to happen? There seems to be a plan of trickery at play. A lying spirit coming through the mouths of Ahab's prophets (ancestor DNA messages), is the plan. Does a lying tongue trigger contaminated cells to become active? Appears so. Taking this another step deeper in thought, messages represent what the cellular records are telling the body. For example: A genetic imprint becomes active, and your body responds to the inflammation or heart disease the genetic record is playing. A form of false messaging has come on the scene because you personally have not encountered a virus (or other means) that would lay the foundation for inflammation or heart disease. Someone in the ancestral line may have had it, OR they lived a lifestyle that after a specific length of time through the generations produced an imprint for inflammation or heart disease. The message playing is not the original but a <u>carbon</u> copy, it's there but not valid in its presentation. This raises another question. Is the chemical element carbon involved in recording the messages that become stuck inside the cells? If a person has a high level of carbon in their body, are they more prone to recording the bad vibes (infections, sounds, etc.) that produce disease down through the generations? Carbon is in all food to some degree and many guidelines for the Elijah Healing and life thereafter have restricted food intake compared to what is normally consumed by a person today. Appears people really do eat themselves unto death.

Previous infections that plagued our ancestors can also come alive in a little different form than the original set of symptoms the ancestor may have experienced. What they experienced as a Herpes related infection may only have an appearance down the generational line as inflammation or cold sores. Speaking a false report or lying causes contamination in the cells or causes pre-existing contamination to come alive. Remember, the title of spirit represents a measure and mysterious mixture of chemical elements. The chemical elements necessary to keep the physical body healthy becomes interrupted or depleted in response to the contaminated genetic imprints. Something that would take a chemist to identify is going on here.

<u>Verses 24-30</u>: These next few verses describe the departure of righteousness. When genetic corruption comes alive, the collection of proper bodily responses and daily required cycles for health departs or becomes overloaded, the "righteousness" leaves. The contaminated DNA, genetic imprints that hold within its very existence the record of disease, must be eliminated from the physical body for the person to meet the requirements that produce righteousness or to be righteous.

Micaiah makes a statement about the act of going into an inner chamber and hiding yourself. For as hard as it is in the days and times we live in, a person must remove themselves from the hustle and bustle of life. Everything that is not vital for your very existence should be eliminated. What do I mean by this? Travel, visiting friends, neighbors or family, attending sporting events or parties, eating outside of the guidelines the Laws have set in place. This includes eating meals away from your home, in restaurants or at dinner parties. Nearly everything considered today to be necessary is not necessary when it comes to cleaning out previously recorded infections or other forms of contamination that reside in your genetic makeup. The body will go through stages of affliction as it eliminates contamination and recalibrates itself. It is not easy to go through but is required if the person is interested in becoming eternal. The hidden DNA code that is identified as Israelite/Israel will eventually show up on your behalf.

<u>Verses 31-40</u>: This Israelite DNA code brings an act of rescue on your behalf. Wounds may come but they will not become deadly if you remain steady in the steps it takes for the cells to be renewed. The inherited genetic corruption will die, but you personally will not die. The scene that is unfolding throughout these verses is eerily similar to the myth of the Phoenix/Firebird. Taking a few minutes to read that myth will help in the interpretation of what is being played out in these verses.

The power of the genetic corruption dies and is laid to rest in a place that is guarded (Samaria) so it cannot rise against you again, unless you fall out of practicing the Laws that govern life.

Dogs are a representation of people who follow the commands of men, the world's systems. Certainly, in this day and time if you become seriously ill it is advised that you seek medical assistance, particularly when you lack the knowledge of how to fight against such things with natural, or you could say spiritual, weapons. Keeping outside intervention at a minimum is a must to stay on the Elijah Healing track. There are certain practices (when to eat, what to eat, when to sleep, how to dress, etc.) that must be followed each day that will remove serious illnesses or diseases but to not do anything in response to such situations could result in a premature trip to the cemetery.

The rest of the events of Ahab's reign and all that he did, including the ivory palace he built, are written in the Book of the Chronicles of the Kings of Israel. So, Ahab rested (slept) with his fathers (ancestors) and Ahaziah (grasp, possession) his son reigned in his place.

<u>Verses 41-54</u>: Jehoshaphat (God has decided) was a son of Asa (to suffer harm; healer or physician) and he began to reign over Judah (notice the specific tribe mentioned) in the *fourth year* of Ahab king of Israel. There were four years of battling cellular corruption handed down from ancestors. Now the story begins to reveal various time frames. First, "God has judged – decided" is connected to 35 years. Could this mean a person must (or will) be 35 years old before they are visited by the Elijah Healing? That would mean there are 35 years of opportunity for the good genes (sin-free cells) to be destroyed, if there are any to be destroyed. Interesting thought. We will keep this in mind as we move along.

The human body was designed to survive. Considering this natural hunger to survive, it appears the world systems are, at times, offering more harm than the physical body can tolerate. The natural cycles of the body are being derailed. Overcrowded physicians' offices and hospitals give testimony to this. A medical intervention may keep you breathing but how healthy are you? What about the number of people that must live their last days under some form of nursing care? Have you visited a local nursing or care home facility? It is a good invitation to weep at the condition of the residents.

Then we are told that this decision of God has dominion over us for 25 years, but this 25-year period resides within Jerusalem, peace. It is beginning to sound like cellular contamination simmers quietly for several years before the encounter with the Elijah Healing process knocks on your door! This might explain why the health of people seems to hit bottom at around 60 years of age. Although today it is becoming more common for 30+ year olds to experience serious health issues. The good genes are dwindling away as time, and generations, move forward.

Jehoshaphat's mother was Azubah (to leave or forsake; desolation) the daughter of Shilhi (to send or let go like firing of an arrow or missile; outstretching; discharge from service). Jehoshaphat lived his life like his father, Asa, who lived according to the Laws that govern life. According to verse 43, there seems to have been a hangup with the burning of incense in what is called "high places."

When Scripture makes a notation that a written record exists in either historical records or a Book of the Chronicles (verse 39), it CAN reference a code within the blood that moves through the generations. A blood code is a record and Jehoshaphat's record has a connection to the line of Judah. Could it be that people who have blood roots in what is called Judah in the bible, have the assignment of tackling the Elijah Healing process that could reach others, others meaning all those who qualify as an "Israelite," through cellular communication? (Remember the brief reference to Ruth and Boaz in Chapter 4?). For those not familiar with cell signaling or cellular communication between persons, this can sound quite foreign. I compare this inner cellular communication ability to that of the use of a cell phone. If you have a person's contact information or cell phone number in your cell phone, at the push of a button or a voice command you can connect with them.

Jehoshaphat does a little housekeeping and removes the remnant of the sodomites (Sodom: deal violently with; destroy + field) both male and female. Sodomites appear to be energetic powers (electricity or possibly magnetism) that cause damage to the body (male is physical;

female is spiritual). A field is not only a plot of ground but also is used to describe a sphere of energy. Jehoshaphat's act of housekeeping removed the ruling power that had been in position over Edom (red. The blood). A lesser authority identified as a deputy served as king.

Ships of Tarshish (white dove or Holy Spirit) were sent to Ophir (Riches, gathering mark for wealth; inner wealth or wisdom) for gold, but something occurred that caused these ships to be broken. Ezion Geber (skeletal structure; strength; backbone of a man). Within these three names, Tarshish, Ophir and Ezion Geber we are told the structure and strength of the spinal cord connects to inner wisdom by way of the Holy Spirit. The crown of the head where the amygdala and pineal glands are placed is a target for the cosmic activities to connect with the human body. When the spinal cord is not functioning properly, there is limited spirit activity that can reach the entirety of the spinal cord.

Jehoshaphat resists the help of Ahaziah (possession) in this wrecked ship situation.

Jehoshaphat dies and joins his ancestors in a state of rest. Jehoshaphat's son Jehoram (Jehovah (owner, master, lord) is exalted) takes his place.

Ahaziah takes a reigning position in Samaria. Again, the verses give specific time-related markers in conjunction to the events that unfold. Ahaziah's position begins in the seventh year of Jehoshaphat's reign as king of Judah. Azaziah is the ruling power of the Israelites for two years. Ahaziah throws things all out of whack by reverting to how his immediate ancestors behaved. Here, Ahaziah represents the activated ancestor corruption that is housed within your DNA. That corruption comes to the surface. Now you could experience a symptom similar to that of your parent(s), exhibit emotions like that of a parent, or any number of other physical manifestations of the pre-recorded information that is floating in your bloodstream. These symptoms can cause a person to seek the advice or treatment from a medical professional and depending upon what that treatment is whether you throw yourself back into a decline in health or whether the treatment was an aid to simply help a person through a time of systemic reactions but did nothing to erase the problem. You still exhibit evidence of the issues experienced prior to taking the steps and spending money on trying to rid them on your own. This type of cycle creates more "sin" within the body. More sin means more suffering and more time to get it cleaned out. God does not respond kindly to seeking outsiders for repair of the physical body.

This scene reminds me of the story of the woman with the issue of blood. She spent all her money on doctors and still had the issue but when she reached out and touched the hem of Jesus's garment, her condition was healed. (Matthew 9:20-22) In this story, Jesus represents the various lifestyle adjustments (Commands) necessary to bring healing to the blood. Uncountable people need to simply take ahold of the hem of His garment.

CHAPTER 7
2 KINGS, CHAPTER 1

IT'S ALL IN YOUR HEAD

<u>Verses 1-8</u>: As if the Israelites didn't have enough going on, these verses reflect issues with the brain in the form of mental health. This is reflected in the meaning of the name Moab: mental; cognitive issues. In Chapter 4 I shared a portion of the story of Ruth and Boaz. Ruth was of the Moabite tribe. This mental health issue seems to appear after the curses left behind by our ancestors have all been shut down, after the death of Ahab. If all the ancestor corruption is removed, what could cause this mental health issue? I inject a little background information here. When God's people strayed from the Laws given to them for keeping not only themselves healthy but also the planet (story of Adam assigned to keeping the garden in tip-top shape), the cosmic activity began to shift in a way that the signals necessary for the human body to function properly, specifically the brain, were diminished. The brain was not being fed like it needed to be. This human initiated cosmic shift is a root cause of many mental health diagnoses seen today. The lack of signals to recharge the brain in one generation then passes to the next generation and so on down the line, eventually burping out a brain that cannot function correctly. Learning issues erupt, sleep issues are on the rise, Bipolar and Schizophrenia become common. The heavens and the creatures that live on the earth become a mess! While the numbers still may be few, there are people who have shifted or are progressively shifting

to a life that brings the cosmic activity back into a favorable position with respect to the human brain. This recovery of the heavens is evident in the display of Northern Lights in locations where they are not normally seen, and spectacular sunrise or sunset scenes. The heavens and the earth are working through their healing phase and in turn, the people on the earth will reap the harvest of it.

Ahaziah (to possess) pulls a Humpty Dumpty act and falls through the lattice of his upper chamber. This chamber was in Samaria (to guard or protect). It appears Ahaziah has a form of protection, accident and recovery insurance policy, maybe, for his decline. Ahaziah sends out messengers to seek information from Baal-zebub (lord of the flies. Flies are drawn to dead things, things that are in the process of decaying). Baal-zebub was the powerful influence that claimed the territory of Ekron (uprooting or extermination). Ekron doesn't sound too promising with that sort of meaning. Ahaziah obviously isn't concerned about what Ekron means, he wants to know if he's going to survive this decline in health he's going through. As previously mentioned, when walking through the Elijah Healing, consulting a healthcare professional instead of consulting God can be risky business. Many treatments or drugs a healthcare professional might suggest conflict with the process the body is attempting to go through to shut down the contaminated genetics.

Meanwhile, Elijah receives a call from an angel telling him to hurry on over to Samaria and inquire if they lack the understanding that God should be consulted about the health issues, not Baal. It would be wise in these situations to not assume you know what God will say about your health situation. Many times, the answer to the problem is far from what you may have been led (or persuaded) to believe. The angel continues with its instructions for Elijah and is quite blunt about the consequences on consulting a Baal, any of them. Here it is, plain and simple: "You will not get up from the sickbed; you will surely die." When you rely on a system or industry for solving a health issue or a form of recovery, chances are high that you will die. The body cannot properly complete its process of elimination of harmful genetics when it is bombarded with such things as chemicals or radiation. Elijah puts on his shoes and takes off to Samaria to deliver the message to the king's messengers. This is when you decide Elijah doesn't have a pleasant job!

The message reaches the king through his messengers, and the king wants to know who this man was that spoke these words. Elijah is described as "a hairy man" (influence; distinctive) who wore a leather belt about his waist (defined midline; dividing point). Ah yes, it was Elijah. Elijah must have a reputation in this town.

<u>Verses 9-15</u>: The king sends his men, 50 at a time, to retrieve Elijah from the hill he was sitting on. Short interpretation here: The Elijah Healing process is in an elevated position (hill). There is a ruling power (king) that is sending groups of 50 captains (leaders) plus 50 men. This would be genetic imprints and/or symptoms that go along with them. For example, initiating infections (captains) and the 50 ancestors (men; men mean the physical body) who carried that infection, or the 50 physical symptoms that infection can present.

Elijah has a little fun with this by calling fire down from heaven to consume the disruptions. By the third round, Elijah is instructed to follow the captain and his men to see the king. These verses describe the Elijah process that remains resident within the head while clusters of 50% of the DNA strands at any one time are eliminated by cosmic activity that consumes the damaged clusters. After two cleansing sessions, the Elijah process remains but lessens in intensity and does not annihilate the harmless inherited DNA strands.

Elijah meets with the king and explains to him why the message he received had a doom and gloom component to it. And, sure enough, Ahaziah died. (Rev. 11:5; 20:9).

<u>Verses 16-18</u>: Elijah is a bit apprehensive but goes to visit the king as instructed. Elijah asks the king, Oh king, did you forget that God will come to your aid when asked? If so, why did you send men to consult with Baal-Zebub?

Elijah continues with the news the king really did not want to hear: Sorry dude, you are going to die in response to your actions.

To be sure everyone is clear about what this is saying: To consult professionals for health-related situations will keep you in your sickbed until your death. You may not die the day you enter the physician's office, but your body will continue in a cycle that eventually plants you at the cemetery. Your job then will be pushing up daisies! Sure enough, the king died according to the word of the Lord.

There is a level of God-given protection that resides within the body when the body is not manipulated, drugged or distracted with various types of physical alterations or exposure. The more prescription drugs, x-rays, radiation exposure, etc. a person goes through, the more the protection decreases. What is that protection? Light filled cells, often received from ancestors several generations prior. Seeking medical intervention can be like having a hole in the bottom of a glass you are attempting to fill with water. Eventually the cup (of light) will run empty. The actions of Ahaziah's life are recorded in the heavens (Book of Chronicles).

What takes place when things are referenced as being recorded in various books? It is a reference to the very acts of the person in a *position of authority while here on earth having planted vibrations that reflect the actions taken within the clouds of the sky, the cosmos. Records are also what pass through the blood to the next generation. In the case of Ahaziah, he authored a genetic code for seeking health-related advice from outsiders, the Baals.*

Now Jehoram (Jehovah is exalted) comes on the scene as the son of Jehoshaphat (God has judged; a position of dealing with consequences, a power that rules over Judah – the ability to praise from an inner-chemistry standpoint) the king of Judah because he had no son (the position of sonship is removed).

CHAPTER 8
2 KINGS, CHAPTER 2

A WHIRLWIND OF ACTIVITY

<u>Verses 1-2</u>: Salvation, in the form of Elisha, has arrived. The Elijah Healing did a great work and now the rescue is in place. The cyclical activity of health issues, decay and disease leaves. This is referenced in Elijah and Elisha leaving Gilgal. The Elijah part of the story is preparing to leave via a whirlwind and Elisha is in place.

During their exit from Gilgal, Elijah tells Elisha to wait at a particular point because the Lord has "sent me to Bethel" (God's house). More easily explained, those who belong to "God's family" will be given the opportunity to clean up the contaminated genetics that is required for becoming an eternal being. Elisha agrees and in his statement of response to Elijah reveals a detail about what happens once a person reaches the point of salvation: As the Lord lives and <u>as your inner being lives</u>, I (Elisha/salvation) shall not leave you. This is a promising statement! Something is going on inside the body that creates a form of life, as in vitality, or abundant life. After the Elijah Healing process is complete, when a person keeps the body in sync with the cosmos, maintains a balance in the chemical elements, salvation (rescue from health dangers) will not leave the body. This is not a card that allows complete and total freedom for a person to eat or live as they please. The Commands/Laws still must be followed to maintain the status reached. A virus or other infection may at some *point afflict you, but it will not overtake you and it will not take up residency within the cells causing the light (photons) to be removed. Cells, DNA, chromosomes and the whole ball of wax in and around them become damaged by infections, stripped of the light (photons). Those damaged quantum particles pass on to the descendants (heirs) burping out disease, disabilities, or syndromes.*

<u>*Verses 3-5*</u>*: While at God's House, Elisha receives some astounding information. There appears to be a form of power lording over the function of the brain (head) and that influential power is scheduled to be removed. Of course, Elisha knows this event was set to unfold. You can't get much past Elisha! Peace is connected to this head-clearing event. These verses connect with the prior Chapters that talk about Moab.*

Elijah is now headed to Jericho (relief + Moon; relief comes through Moon phases directed to the head) and tells Elisha to stay put. Elisha is not keen on separating from Elijah so the two of them travel to Jericho. Now in Jericho, Elisha receives the same message he did in Bethel. He is told that the Lord will take his master away. Whatever is lording over Elisha or has been the master of what he represents is obviously known in a few communities. There is a type of brain signal interruption that is about to be corrected.

The journey continues and Elijah and Elisha travel to the Jordan (Jordan means down under, as a reference to inside the body).

<u>*Verses 6-10*</u>*: Verse 7 references 50 men. A logical meaning to this "50 men" would be ancestor imprints. Using the word men as a reference to the physical and 50 as a reference to 50%, it is possible that half of what is being addressed in the blood is from the male's (father) ancestors and the other half would be from the female's (mother)*

ancestors. It appears there is something on the interior of the body, unrelated to genetic imprints, that is causing friction with Elijah and Elisha. Could this friction be something that happens when a person classified as an Israelite has children with a person classified as "foreign"? Two different types of gene components that mesh together and the result upsets brain function in the descendants. (See, Overview).

In the previous verses there is a reference of the moon (Jericho). As discussed, signals that originate through cosmic activity are important for proper brain function. Would these few verses be an indication that the other half of healing the body is the restoration of the cosmic signals the brain needs? If salvation is restricted when the proper cosmic signaling is not available, this tells me no human being as reached "salvation" for a very long time. Whatever the case, there is a stand-off between these 50 that reside "down under," the Elijah Healing and salvation.

Elijah uses his powerful tools and strikes the waters and divides them. The water, in this case, would be blood plasma. The act of dividing reflects the blood and the plasma separating. The inherited disruptive imprints that had taken up residence in the blood are now cast out through the act of the body reducing its water/plasma. Just like a stream, when the water dries up, so do the bacteria, fungi or other micro-organisms. After the stream bed is completely dried and all harmful disruptions are gone, the waters will fill the blood once again. This act of drying takes place inside the body and unfolds during the season of summer with the act of refilling taking place in the spring, Nisan. Sadly, the belief that the body must have "x" ounces of water each day is over-stepping boundaries put in place by nature. The more $H2O$ a person drinks, the harder it is for the body to reduce the volume of water. Over consumption of water can interrupt the natural process of drying up the rivers inside our body and allowing the infections to die off.

Elijah is preparing to depart and asks Elisha if he has any final requests of him. Elisha gives an interesting response stating that he desired a <u>double portion</u>, indicating he wants twice as much of the spirit that has been resident in and upon Elijah. Once the Elijah Healing is complete and salvation has been obtained, salvation provides a double protection for the body.

<u>Verses 11-14</u>: Elijah and Elisha continue their stroll and discuss the events they have experienced when suddenly, through a powerful cleansing act, the two were separated and the Elijah Healing returned to the cosmos. (Rev. 11:12).

Elisha witnesses this event and he cried, My father. My father! The chariot of Israel and its horsemen! Then he saw him no more and he took hold of his own clothes and tore them into two pieces. Clothing is symbolic of whatever is on the inside will come forth to the outside. Clothing provides an exterior statement about a person's status. Tearing the clothing into two pieces can tell us that there is a two-part process to what is called salvation. This two-part process is seen in the contamination that alters genes being collected by the plasma and then the plasma being reduced to nothing to kill off the contamination. The second part comes from the activity of the cosmos that maintains healthy brain function. The human body can be detoxed, disinfected, flushed, energized and realigned but without the assistance of the cosmic activity, those manmade efforts can only bring 50% of a desired healthy outcome. The remainder is "up to God."

Elisha being in a state of shock grabs Elijah's mantle and prayer shawl and heads to the Jordan (down under). The salvation of every individual takes place in the blood. When the blood is clean of genetic imprints and the daily and weekly practices are in place to keep it clean, there is salvation. Salvation remains active with the aid of the cosmic signals that reach the human body via the brain. Salvation does not come through a printed or verbal prayer.

<u>Verses 15-18</u>: Elisha encounters some of the individuals from his prior Jericho visit and they recognize the essence (energetic influence) that Elijah had now resting upon Elisha. These men give a sign of submission to the power that Elisha is now carrying and bow before him. This scene tells us that a physical encounter (infection) will bow when a person carries a status of salvation. The infection will not take up residence.

The act of an actual bow becomes important. This bow is to be done in the form of what is known in yoga as a child's pose. This simple forehead to the floor pose provides a form of protection to the brain, an act of equalizing the contents of the head. The bow is important prior to laying down for sleep and upon rising for the day to assist in the transition of the head from being vertical to being horizontal and vice versa.

The men ask Elisha if 50 of the strong men should go out and search for the master that once ruled over Elisha. Let's stop here for a moment. What could have been or currently does rule over the truth about salvation? The answer that comes to my mind is religions. Religion has handed out a different definition and set of requirements for salvation than what the bible teaches. How do I know this? Because I've experienced and become familiar with both. Saying a prayer with or without the accompaniment of a person in a position of authority within a religion or not does little or nothing for rescuing the body from disease. Rescuing the body from disease is salvation. The bible teaches salvation although it has not been taught with respect to the health of the physical body. How do I know the standard "prayer of salvation" is nothing but a mouth full of words? Because 99.9% of the earth's population who have recited the "prayer of salvation" is still carrying around grandma's kidney disease, or grandpa's crooked spine, or great grandma's bad teeth, and so forth. When there is salvation as taught by Jesus, the inherited diseases are no longer present. You have been rescued from the curses cast upon you by your ancestors.

The 50 men show up on the scene once again and present the suggestion of finding Elijah. Where did Elijah go? Did the Spirit of the Lord simply take him away to some unknown destination? The reference to mountain and valley in these verses could be a reference to meridian points in the body. It is clear that the Elijah Healing process is no longer needed once a person reaches Elisha, salvation.

Elisha is not convinced that searching for Elijah is a good idea and advises against it. Once the status of salvation is achieved, there is no need to return to an Elijah Healing process. Maintenance is important but a full-blown Elijah Healing process is unnecessary. The 50 continue nagging at Elisha and Elisha gives in to the pressure. Ok, go ahead. Three days pass, and Elijah is nowhere to be found. Here's when Elisha says, "I told you so."

<u>Verses 19-22</u>: Things become peaceful although some issues are still in need of a little repair. The plasma is still going through its cleansing process, which can take a few months. Growth has ceased in the form of cells taking a sabbatical from their normal cycles. Things have sort of stalled out. The Elijah Healing process has brought peace (versus the health chaos created by contaminated genes) but the process must be applied by each individual so the plasma becomes clean and

descendants can prosper. When the plasma is contaminated, the contamination passes through to, and becomes a part of, a developing fetus. Basically, a developing child swims in contaminated water for 9 months. And we wonder where birth defects come from!

Salt is key in healing the plasma. Notice the reference to spring of water and the salt. A spring of water moves, is active. Motionless fluids do not seem to benefit from the salt whereas fluids that move within the body do. Salt supplies a form of cleansing as a person moves forward from the completion of the Elijah Healing. As stated in verses 21 and 22: "No longer will death or unfruitfulness result from it" ("it" being dirty plasma). "Therefore, the water remains healthy to this very day…" I strongly suggest eating sea salt. Table salt is good for rinsing the mouth or using with baking soda for a scouring powder but table salt does nothing for keeping the plasma healthy and clean.

<u>Verses 23-25</u>: Elisha sets out to God's House. During his journey he encounters some young men (some translations say small boys) who had come from the city. These young men appear to be well versed in mocking or teasing. I'm sure Elisha was a bit annoyed by their taunting. These young men mention Elisha having a bald head. Balding is one symptom of the Elijah Healing process. As the body moves through the various stages required to eliminate genetic imprints, thinning hair, bald spots or even change in hair texture can become evident. This seemingly minor issue makes me wonder if the numerous bald heads present in the world today are a result of the body attempting to go through the Elijah Healing process and due to the lack of knowledge on behalf of the person on how to maneuver through the process, the hair falls out but the Elijah Healing is never completed. This would leave a genetic imprint for balding. There are other factors that can play into thinning hair or balding for sure.

Rest assured, if the hair begins to fall out during the Elijah Healing, once the healing process is complete, new hair will grow. To minimize the loss of hair, use the tips of the fingers and massage the scalp for a few minutes daily.

Hair acts as an antenna and has a form of electrical attraction that draws the signals present in the cosmos. These signals are necessary for the proper electrical function of the meridians and has an impact on the overall function of the body. The moon presents powerful energy interaction with the brain, and the hair plays an important role in the attraction, distribution and filtration of those energies. A bald head has a risk of too much cosmic energy collecting in the head which can result in brain cancers or electrical interference within the brain. This electrical situation also presents a question of whether it is safe to wear the hair in a bun or other form of collection on the head. The answer to this would need to be on a case-by-case basis. In most cases I would say it is safe to wear the hair in a bun or similar fashion on occasion. I certainly would not support a bun in the hair on a daily basis.

Additional insight on the subject continues through the last few verses.

Verse 24 mentions two female bears that come out of the woods. These she bears mauled "forty-two children." When children are mentioned in a manner such as this, it is referencing descendants. Wood represents a family tree. A form of powerful, devastating injury comes at the descendants.

The number 42 relates to the bladder meridian that runs along the back. This verse may be an indication of injuries related to the bladder and/or gallbladder. Wilderness or woods can be connected to the gallbladder meridian in the top of the foot.

Elisha goes to Mount Carmel (garden; the Wilderness Mound is a gallbladder meridian, and the Big Mound is a meridian for the pericardium), and from there he returned to Samaria (to guard). Guard what has been given you through the Elijah Healing process. A garden, as referenced in the meaning for Mount Carmel, is a symbol of things that grow and mature, becoming a benefit to the body; where seeds are planted and take root. This is seen in the activity of cell replication after the Elijah Healing process is complete. A garden is also a symbol of fresh plant foods such as fruits, squash, vegetables. I advise eating an abundance of fresh fruit in its season during and after the Elijah Healing process.

CHAPTER 9

RAINING MANNA

The Elijah Healing will bring many changes to the body with many symptoms and signs as it progresses. During my studies for this publication, I discovered that the term manna is a reference to the mouth by way of the breath and the electrical activity that comes through the teeth. Strange, but true. I'll help you connect the dots that accommodate this conclusion.

In Hebrew manna means portion, generosity or gift. Manna is said to <u>fall with the dew that fell during the night</u>.

I don't want to get too far off course here but notice the word gift as a meaning for manna? Gifts are connected to Christmas time, December, when oddly enough Santa, dressed in a red suit (red reflects blood; an influence to the blood that comes from the heavens), flies through the air to distribute gifts. Are you following me? We may stumble onto the true origins of the current day Christmas story if we keep going. Another gift receiving day is a person's birthday. This will take some additional study time so for now I strongly suggest that a gift of manna comes to a person in December near Christmas, and at their yearly birthday. Two important manna-gift dates. I also suspect that Hannukah and Diwali must be a part of this manna distribution as well. These dates are important to know because there are qualifications to be met before having the ability to receive. Sounds like Santa's naughty or nice list! Interesting.

Numbers 11:6-7, 9 (HCS): But now our appetite is gone; there's nothing to look at but this manna! The manna resembled coriander seed, and its appearance was like that of bdellium. (Bdellium is tree resin, similar to myrrh.)

9: When the dew fell on the camp at night, the manna would fall with it (cosmic activity producing or activating chemical elements that drop to the earth during nighttime hours). Moses heard the people, family after family (generations), crying at the entrance of their tents (could entrance be a reference to the mouth?). The Lord was very angry; Moses was also provoked. (Things get stirred up.)

An opportunity arises for generations of imprints to begin to stir, causing disruptions in the body. This interpretation is pulled from the references to complain, family after family, crying and anger in the verse above.

A google search provided the following information on coriander seed:

> Coriander seeds are rich in various organic compounds, primarily essential oils with linalool (a terpene alcohol) being the most abundant, alongside significant amounts of y-terpinene, a-pinene, camphor and geraniol, which contribute to its distinct aroma. Beyond these volatile compounds coriander also contains nutritional elements like protein, fiber, fats, vitamins (C, K, A), minerals (calcium, iron, potassium, magnesium), flavonoids, phenolics, fatty acids and sterols making them a versatile spice and nutraceutical.

Obviously, this nutritional information was unknown to the people of the time in which the Scripture was written. The coriander seed information tells us that when a person transitions from the world's systems to and through the Elijah Healing process, and for the remainder of their days eat, in today's terms, limited foods, the chemical elements from the heavens (noted as coriander seeds) provide many nutrients that are necessary for the physical body. A person becomes, you could say, fed by the Spirit. (Matthew 4:4)

Manna has a connection to the jaw/mouth, as an entrance point, with the teeth playing a specific role in electricity. The teeth activate the chemical elements by means of the electrical system that is present in teeth and that electrical activity is necessary for functions of the brain and other organs. Could the elements, coming in contact with the electricity from the teeth, cause the production of nutrients like those found in coriander seeds? Saliva would have a role in this as well. When teeth are drilled, bleached, removed, filled, crowned or capped the value of the tooth function is depleted and eventually comprehension and retention of information will be hindered.

Taking this another step further, since the water/plasma is in a state of increase and decrease to wash away unwanted debris, and rain is only abundant in certain seasons, is this picture of events showing us that a healthy body is reliant upon fluctuations in nutrient intake, depending upon the season? This presents a situation where, for example only, the body needs more protein during Spring (rainy season) than it does in the other three seasons. It appears the body just might be healthier if we toss out the daily multi-vitamin and mineral supplements! The cosmos will regulate the nutrition needed.

Various verses in the bible refer to teeth as fangs, iron, spears or swords. Something important is going on with the teeth. <u>Psalm 58:6</u>: God, knock the teeth out of their mouths; Lord, tear out the young lion's fangs. (HCS). Sounds like if there is a desire to injure someone, the teeth are a good place to start!

Thanks to the dental industry (and they are not the only industry to thank) most people suffer some form of interruption to good health. Manna is not something that is seen but rather a chemical element (or elements) that is received during the nighttime hours, during sleep. This chemical element combo seems to be attracted through the mouth and makes contact with the teeth. For the best manna result during the Elijah Healing, it is advised to avoid all forms of dental work as much as possible. Avoiding all forms of work done to the head or neck is also advised.

<u>John 6:31 (HCS)</u>: Our fathers (ancestors) ate the manna in the wilderness, just as it is written: He gave them bread from heaven to eat. (Carbon, hydrogen and oxygen atoms are found in wheat.)

<u>Psalm 78:24 (HCS)</u>: He rained manna for them to eat; He gave them grain from heaven.

Teeth play an important role in the receiving of cosmic signals and distributing electrical pulses to the various organs in the body. A Tooth Meridian Chart will show the various organs influenced by each tooth.

<u>Deuteronomy 8:3, 16 (HCS)</u>: He humbled you by letting you go hungry; then He gave you manna to eat, which you and your fathers had not known, so that you might learn that man does not live on bread alone but on every word that comes from the mouth of the

Lord. <u>16</u>: *He fed you in the wilderness with manna that your fathers had not known in order to humble and test you, so that in the end He might cause you to prosper.*

The Elijah Healing is a humbling experience. Giving up foods that have been on the menu since childhood or even those that are reported to be good for the body can be challenging. Calorie intake is slashed to allow toxic cells to die-off. Vitamin and mineral intake are nothing compared to the requirement guidelines for nutrients that have been reported. There are days you wonder how the body can recover or even function when nutritional intake is teetering on slim margins. How? By the chemical elements (breath/words) that come from the cosmos, the manna. When the elements are allowed to be in greater measure than food, and nutrients from those foods, the elements perform their magic. I compare this combination of elements with the aid of electrical pulses to the Holy Spirit. It is as though the Holy Spirit takes control, breathing life back into the body, resurrecting the ancient healthy genetics the body was designed to have and maintain, and bringing life to the mere vessel we use to commute through life on earth called the physical body.

In Deuteronomy 8:16, the words "so that in the end He might cause you to prosper" is speaking of the end of your physical life when all is said and done and you are ready to escape the body and be present with the Lord. The word prosper connects to how the body will be healthy and ultimately the soul will be healthy as well. This conclusion goes with <u>3 John 1:2</u>: *Beloved I pray that you prosper AND be in health EVEN AS thy soul prospers.* The physical body must be healthy first, then the soul will be healthy. The Elijah Healing heals the body and the soul follows.

<u>Nehemiah 9:20 (HCS)</u>: You sent Your good Spirit to instruct them (provided wisdom). You did not withhold Your manna from their mouths, and You gave them water (Living Water) for their thirst.

The correct combination of chemical elements will deliver wisdom. That wisdom will walk you through the Elijah Healing. The chemical elements work with and through the mouth, the entrance to the body, to provide the necessary nutrition. Add hydrogen from fresh bread to the oxygen being taken in through the breath and the body will produce the hydration necessary for the various cycles it goes through to keep the body clean.

<u>Revelation 2:17 (NKJ)</u>: He who has an ear let him hear what the Spirit says to the churches; To him that overcomes (has success through the Elijah Healing) will I give some of the hidden manna (cosmic activity that brings the chemical elements, connecting with the electrical pulses from the teeth, causing an influence to the blood), and will give him a white stone (eternal), a new name written on the stone which no one knows except the one who receives it.

White stones are symbolic of purity and eternity. Stones also represent things that are not easily changed or moved. White stone is a reference to your identity becoming eternal. You become an eternal being once you move through the Elijah Healing with success, receive the Elisha salvation and abide by the limitations necessary to keep the body in proper order. (Revelation 3:5; Luke 10:20)

This verse may shed some light on how the Greeks and Romans followed the myths about gods and goddesses. An eternal figure that receives a heavenly name. The eternal name is written and fixed in place for all time.

The Elijah Healing process is the wilderness experience spoken of in Exodus, Chapters 13-15. When a person is removed from the worldly systems and industries (Egypt), their body will go through a type of weaning process. The body must, and will if given the proper circumstances, adjust to lower calorie intake, have the ability to convert chemical elements to a recipe that is suitable and beneficial for the body, begin its natural cleaning cycle that prevents infection from taking up residence within the cells and in turn, eliminating inherited infections that lead to disease. Using a worldly system to attempt to address a health-related illness or disease is not eliminating the underlying fire (often an infection) that is causing the problem. A remedy from the worldly systems may stomp out the fire for a period of time, but the issue will remain in a smoldering state and will, one day in the future, ignite into a blazing inferno.

Moses led the people through the wilderness for 40 years. Does this equate to a person moving through their wilderness experience for 40 years? I hope not. At this point, there is not a sufficient answer for that question. Personally, I had numerous health crises for most of my life to date. Did I know through those years that I needed the Elijah Healing to remove the cycle of poor health? Not at all. This insight was lost over time, hidden deep in the past. Approaching the health issues I had experienced with a worldly system remedy would cause a negative kick-back in my body. To realize the well-accepted and often popular systems were contributing to the health disruptions took several years. What must take place to reach lasting good health is removing oneself from the worldly system(s), the Baals, and advancing to a life of living with the Spirit Energy (cosmic activity). Some will die in their wilderness experience, in part due to the lack of knowledge of how to escape the cyclical health crisis they experience, and another part will be due to sheer stubbornness. For some, stepping into an Elijah Healing process and throwing aside their current world system remedies would be nothing but suicide. Their body is too far along a world system path to have the ability to turn around and move in the opposite direction.

By sharing my story, it is my hope that the cycles of health crisis, diseases that are present from the point of birth (more likely conception), and crippling conditions related to cellular interruptions will become minimized or, better yet, cease.

CONCLUSION

The Elijah Healing process is equivalent to the cleansing of sin as described in the story of Jesus. Elijah, like Jesus, holds a position of mediator between heaven (cleansing the plasma through the correlation of Heavenly Gases – chemical elements) and man (the physical body). In part, Elijah correlates the electrical activity present in the clean plasma that attracts and is fueled with Heavenly Gases giving life to the meridians (highways). The role of Elijah is a display of what takes place on the interior of the physical body while the role of Jesus displays what can take place on the exterior of the body (i.e., you will feel like you are being whipped at times when a genetic imprint comes alive and you experience the replay of the original virus, bacteria, etc. People will question the periods of isolation that are necessary for the body to recalibrate. And people may accuse you of being influenced by Baal-Zebub, the prince of demons, when they learn of the lifestyle choices and changes you have made!)

It is key, as stated before, to remain vigilant. Do not waiver in any detail that is required for a successful journey through the Elijah Healing. Having a voice of support will assist in successfully making your way through days of extreme fatigue or times of hunger. Keep in mind the prize at the end of the journey. Eternal Life.

Izauh 61®

RESOURCES

Holy Bible:
Holman Christian Standard
New King James Version

Suggested Reading:

From AntiChrist to I AM
Food for the Journey to I AM
    Published 2022, Harvest of Healing, LLC
Home-Made Answers for Cancer and Life Altering Disease
    Published 2024, Harvest of Healing, LLC
Living by the Light of the Moon
    Published 2024, Harvest of Healing, LLC
Eating Yourself to Death
    Published 2024, Harvest of Healing, LLC
The Powerful Influence of Clothing: Color, Fabric, Style
    Published 2025, Harvest of Healing, LLC
Healing the Heart – A Story of King David
    Published 2025, Harvest of Healing, LLC

www.ingramcontent.com/pod-product-compliance
Lightning Source LLC
Chambersburg PA
CBHW020249010526
44107CB00002B/166